TREATING DEPRESSION WITH EMDR THERAPY

Arne Hofmann, MD, PhD, is a specialist in psychosomatic and internal medicine, director of the EMDR Institute, and senior physician of the Gezeiten Haus Clinic for Psychosomatics, Psychotraumatology, and EMDR in Schloss Eichholz (Wesseling). He introduced the EMDR method in Germany in 1991 and is co-founder and honorary member of the German-speaking professional society for psychotraumatology (DeGPT) and the professional societies for EMDR Europe and EMDRIA Germany. He researches and teaches internationally in the field of treatment of trauma sequelae and depression. He has been awarded international prizes and the Federal Cross of Merit for his work.

Luca Ostacoli, MD, is a psychiatrist. He is professor of clinical psychology at the University of Turin, Department of Clinical and Biological Sciences, School of Medicine and Surgery; head of the Clinical and Psychosomatic Psychology Service at S. Luigi Hospital (Orbassano, Turin, from 2001 to 2016); on the Clinical Obstetric Gynecological Psychology Service (from 2016 to present); and on the Psychotraumatology and Health Staff Support Service (City of Health and Science Hospital of Turin from 2019 to present). He is a member of the International Research Consortia and author of numerous scientific publications in the field of trauma-focused interventions, EMDR, and Mindfulness and their neurobiological correlates. He is co-founder of the academic spin-off MindToMove (www.mindtomove .it). He is a psychotherapist with body dynamics training. He is an EMDR Supervisor and Trainer in Clinical Mindfulness and Sensorimotor Psychotherapy, and conducts training seminars on psychotherapy. In 2018, he was awarded the EMDR International Association Award and in 2019 the Francine Shapiro Award from EMDR Europe.

Maria Lehnung, PhD, is a psychological psychotherapist, did research at the University of Kiel with a neurobiological focus, and is now in private practice with a psychotraumatological focus. In addition, she is active as a lecturer and supervisor and EMDR Europe trainer. From the beginning of her work with EMDR, she was fascinated by the procedure and its possibilities and interested in finding creative ways of using EMDR even with difficult patients. For years she has been involved in the scientific research of EMDR therapy and was instrumental in developing the concept of treating depression with EMDR.

Michael Hase, MD, PhD, is a psychiatrist and psychotherapist and director of the Lüneburg Center for Stress Medicine. After his training in neurology and psychiatry, he worked as a senior physician at the Psychiatric Hospital in Lüneburg in Lower Saxony State, where he established the treatment focus on psychotraumatology. He then headed departments for psychosomatic rehabilitation and psychotherapy in Hamburg and Bad Bevensen and is the head physician of the rehabilitation clinic Therapeutischer Hof Toppenstedt. Alongside Arne Hofmann, Hase provided decisive impetus for starting research into depression treatment with EMDR therapy. He teaches and publishes internationally and was awarded the 2018 Outstanding Research Award by the EMDR International Association (EMDRIA) professional society for his work.

Marilyn Luber, PhD, is a licensed, clinical psychologist in private practice in Philadelphia. She was on the Founding Board of Directors of EMDRIA and a member of the EMDR Task Force for Dissociative Disorders. She has conducted training both nationally and internationally and is a co-facilitator for the EMDR Global Alliance. She is on the Steering Committee for the Future of EMDR Therapy Project, on the Council of Scholars, and chair of the "What Is EMDR?" working group. She received HAP's Humanitarian Services Award (1997), Outstanding Contribution to EMDRIA Award (2003), and EMDRIA's Francine Shapiro Award (2005). In 2001, HAP published *Handbook for EMDR Clients* translated into eight languages. She edited seven books for Springer's EMDR Scripted Protocol series. She co-authored Dr. Shapiro's 2009 interview for the *Journal of EMDR Practice and Research* and wrote Dr. Shapiro's 2015 entry for E. S. Neukrug's *The SAGE Encyclopedia of Theory in Counseling and Psychotherapy*. In 2020, she edited a free-access resource, EMDR Resources in the Era of COVID-19 (https://marilynluber.files.wordpress.com/2020/06/emdr-resources-for-covid.pdf).

TREATING DEPRESSION WITH EMDR THERAPY

Techniques and Interventions

Arne Hofmann, MD, PhD

Luca Ostacoli, MD

Maria Lehnung, PhD

Michael Hase, MD, PhD

Marilyn Luber, PhD

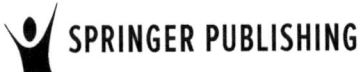

Copyright © 2023 Springer Publishing Company, LLC
All rights reserved.

No part of this publication may be reproduced, stored in a retrieval system, or transmitted in any form or by any means, electronic, mechanical, photocopying, recording, or otherwise, without the prior permission of Springer Publishing Company, LLC, or authorization through payment of the appropriate fees to the Copyright Clearance Center, Inc., 222 Rosewood Drive, Danvers, MA 01923, 978-750-8400, fax 978-646-8600, info@copyright.com or at www.copyright.com.

Springer Publishing Company, LLC
11 West 42nd Street, New York, NY 10036
www.springerpub.com
connect.springerpub.com/

Acquisitions Editor: Kate Dimock
Compositor: Transforma

ISBN: 978-0-8261-3965-8
ebook ISBN: 978-0-8261-3966-5
DOI: 10.1891/9780826139665

Printed by LSI

The author and the publisher of this Work have made every effort to use sources believed to be reliable to provide information that is accurate and compatible with the standards generally accepted at the time of publication. The author and publisher shall not be liable for any special, consequential, or exemplary damages resulting, in whole or in part, from the readers' use of, or reliance on, the information contained in this book. The publisher has no responsibility for the persistence or accuracy of URLs for external or third-party Internet websites referred to in this publication and does not guarantee that any content on such websites is, or will remain, accurate or appropriate.

Library of Congress Cataloging-in-Publication Data
LCCN: 2022014885

Contact sales@springerpub.com to receive discount rates on bulk purchases.

Publisher's Note: **New and used products purchased from third-party sellers are not guaranteed for quality, authenticity, or access to any included digital components.**

Printed in the United States of America.

Contents

Contributors   ix
Acknowledgments   xi

Introduction to Treating Depression With EMDR Therapy   1
Arne Hofmann

PART I: MEMORY WORK—A NEW METHOD FOR THE TREATMENT OF DEPRESSION: EMDR THERAPY

1. EMDR Therapy as a New Treatment Approach   **23**
   Maria Lehnung and Michael Hase

PART II: THE EMDR DeprEnd TREATMENT MANUAL

2. The EMDR Protocol for the Treatment of Depression (DeprEnd)   **39**
   Michael Hase

3. Preparation and Stabilization in EMDR Therapy for Depressive Patients   **53**
   Luca Ostacoli, Sara Carletto, Carmen Settanta, Lorena Giovinazzo, and Francesca Malandrone

4. Processing Episode Triggers With EMDR Therapy   **97**
   Arne Hofmann

5. Treating Belief Systems With EMDR Therapy   **109**
   Maria Lehnung

6. Processing Depressive or Suicidal States With EMDR Therapy   **121**
   Michael Hase

7. Relapse Prevention With EMDR Therapy **129**
   Maria Lehnung

8. Comorbidity With Complex Trauma-Related Disorders and EMDR Therapy **137**
   Arne Hofmann, Susanne Altmeyer, and Visal Tumani

9. The EMDR-Drawing Integration (EMDR-DI) Protocol: A Visual Approach to Complex Posttraumatic Stress Disorder, Dissociation, and Depressive States **145**
   Gabriella Bertino, Luca Ostacoli, Sara Carletto, and Francesca Malandrone

PART III: FUTURE PERSPECTIVES OF EMDR THERAPY

10. The State of Research and Practical Experience on Treating Bipolar Disorder With EMDR Therapy **171**
    Benedikt L. Amann

11. Traumatic Events and Severe Recurrent and Chronic Depression and EMDR Therapy: Clinical and Biological Issues **183**
    Alessandra Minelli and Elisabetta Maffioletti

12. Consequences for Practical Work With EMDR Therapy **195**
    Arne Hofmann and Marilyn Luber

PART IV: RESOURCES

13. Randomized Controlled Scientific Studies on EMDR and Depression **201**
    Sara Carletto, Francesca Malandrone, and Luca Ostacoli

14. How to Fill the Symptom Event Map **205**
    Arne Hofmann

15. Finding a Certified EMDR Therapist **209**
    Marilyn Luber and Arne Hofmann

Index 211

Contributors

Susanne Altmeyer, MD, is a specialist in psychosomatic medicine and head physician of the Gezeiten Haus Clinic for Psychosomatics, Psychotraumatology, and EMDR in Schloss Eichholz (Wesseling). One of her main areas of expertise is the combination of systemic therapy and EMDR therapy, especially for trauma sequelae and depression.

Benedikt L. Amann, MD, is a psychiatrist, psychotherapist, and senior researcher at the Consortium Parc de Salut Mar and the Hospital del Mar Medical Research Institute, Barcelona, and also an associate professor at the Autonomous University of Barcelona. His research focuses on the prevalence of psychological trauma in psychiatric conditions, on EMDR as a therapeutic approach focused on trauma in the psychiatric setting, and on mental well-being and health in the workplace. He regularly presents at national and international conferences and has more than 110 PubMed indexed publications.

Gabriella Bertino, PhD, is a psychologist and relational systemic psychotherapist. She is a specialist in psychotraumatology and relational mindfulness and an EMDR Italy consultant. She collaborates in research on EMDR and Clinical Mindfulness and lectures in master's courses at the Department of Clinical and Biological Sciences of the University of Turin.

Sara Carletto, PhD, is a psychologist, and psychotherapist, with her PhD in neuroscience and training in Clinical Mindfulness and trauma-focused therapies. She is an EMDR practitioner and researcher in Clinical Psychology at the Department of Neuroscience, "Rita Levi Montalcini" of the University of Turin, School of Medicine and Surgery. She works at the Psychology Service of the Sant'Anna Obstetric Gynecological Hospital of the City of Health and Science Hospital of Turin. She is a member of the academic spin-off MindToMove (www.mindtomove.it). She is involved in clinical psychological research on the efficacy, mechanisms of action, and neurobiological effects of psychological and psychotherapeutic treatments such as EMDR therapy and mindfulness-based interventions. She received awards from the EMDR International Association (Outstanding Contribution to Research, 2018) and from EMDR Europe (Francine Shapiro Award, 2019) for her research.

Lorena Giovinazzo, PhD, is a psychologist, cognitive psychotherapist, clinical sexologist, and EMDR practitioner. She has training in Mindfulness, and collaborates on research projects with the Department of Clinical and Biological Sciences and with the Department of Neuroscience of the University of Turin, with the academic spin-off MindToMove, and with the Clinical Psychology Service, City of Health and Science Hospital of Turin.

Elisabetta Maffioletti, PhD, is a biologist and postdoctoral research associate in the field of biology psychiatric disorders in the Department of Molecular and Translational Medicine, Subdepartment of Biology and Genetics, University of Brescia, Italy.

Francesca Malandrone, PhD, is a psychologist and student in experimental medicine at the University of Turin, with Cognitive Constructivist Relational and Mindfulness training. She collaborates in Didactics and Research with the Department of Clinical and Biological Sciences, with the academic spin-off MindToMove, and with the Clinical Psychology Service, AOU City of Health and Science of Turin.

Alessandra Minelli, PhD, is professor of psychobiology in the Department of Molecular and Translational Medicine, Subdepartment of Biology and Genetics, at the University of Brescia, Italy. She teaches and publishes internationally.

Carmen Settanta, PhD, is a psychologist and psychotherapist. Her degree is in neuroscience, and she has had training in Cognitive Constructivist Relational therapy, EMDR, and Mindfulness. She collaborates with the Department of Clinical and Biological Sciences of the University of Turin.

Visal Tumani, MD, is a specialist in psychiatry and psychotherapy in the psychiatric department III of the University of Ulm. She has been researching and publishing for many years in the field of neurobiology and application of EMDR therapy in complex trauma sequelae, in depressive disorders, and in patients with a migration background.

Acknowledgments

A book such as this cannot be written by a single author. Instead, it was written by a group of curious clinicians and researchers determined to better treat the chronic suffering of their depressed patients and clients. Some among this group are included in the list of coauthors, but a number of others are not.

At this point, we would first like to thank our colleagues and friends at the EMDR Institute Germany, who supported us in our first retrospective study more than 10 years ago and thus helped us to find the first systematic evidence for the effectiveness of EMDR therapy with depressed patients.

Our thanks also go to the professional society for EMDR in Germany that supported us in our first controlled study at a time when it was still unclear what the results would be. Equal thanks go to EMDR Europe, that also supported our studies by giving us the opportunities to establish ourselves as an EDEN research group at the 2010 European Conference in Hamburg, and later to continue meeting at the European conferences.

Further thanks go to Isabel Fernandez and the Italian EMDR professional society and all the colleagues involved in this project.

A special thanks goes to our Italian friends in Turin and to the team of Anabel Gonzalez in A Coruña, Spain. Without your great efforts to conduct our first international EDEN RCT study, we would not have been able to conduct the equivalence study on EMDR and behavior therapy.

Publishing a book by many authors, such as this one, is a complex task. Thanks to Springer Publishing Company, our American publisher, and our acquisitions editor, Kate Dimock, with the support of Kirsten Elmer, assistant editor. A special thanks to David Nelson, who translated our book from German into English, and Marilyn Luber, who translated the Academic German translation into a more colloquial, yet professional, version for our work.

An extra big thank you goes to the EMDR Foundation, that supported us with $25,000 at a time when we urgently needed this for the completion of the first international EDEN study.

We would also like to thank the research team of Professor Benedikt Amann in Barcelona, head of the Centro Fòrum research unit within the Parc de Salut Mar, associated with the Autonomous University of Barcelona, IMIM and CIBERSAM, Madrid.

Similarly, our thanks also go to Professor Alessandra Minnelli and her team from the Department of Molecular and Translational Medicine at the University of Brescia in Italy.

A very special thank you also belongs to our partners who have supported us during the writing of this book, even though this has cost valuable family time.

Finally, but with special emphasis, we would like to express our great gratitude to our patients and clients. They were open to treatment with EMDR therapy and their open-mindedness and feedback enabled us to find out which interventions helped and which were less helpful. This book was written to enable other clinicians and researchers to continue research and learning in this area and to develop better treatments for future generations of depressed patients.

Introduction to Treating Depression With EMDR Therapy

Arne Hofmann

INTRODUCTION

This book introduces a new, successful, research-based, and proven approach to treat depressive disorders. In this introduction, we give an overview of the successes and limitations of current guideline-based treatment of depressive disorders as well as an overview of our 12 years of research in this field. We found that an approach that considers depression as a stress- and trauma-based disorder is critical for treating depressive patients, especially patients who do not respond well to current guideline-based treatment. Eye movement desensitization and reprocessing (EMDR) therapy is the centerpiece of this new treatment and has already shown its effectiveness in treating depression successfully in a number of controlled studies. This book contains many case studies and information to inform the practice of EMDR-trained clinicians.

HISTORY OF TREATING DEPRESSION WITH EMDR THERAPY

This book was written by an international group of clinicians and researchers who have been studying the treatment of depressive disorders with EMDR therapy collectively for over 10 years. At the time of this book's publication, we have conducted five controlled clinical studies about this treatment, including three randomized controlled trial (RCT) studies. In addition, we have treated over 800 depressive patients using the conclusions gained from this research (Hase et al., 2015, 2018; Minelli et al., 2019; Ostacoli et al., 2018). These findings have led to the development of an approach for treating depressive disorders that we introduce in this book.

Central to our new approach is the observation that most depressive disorders are related to stressful life experiences. These experiences seem to result in specific memory changes that are closely linked to depressive symptoms. These structures of memory, which we call pathogenic memories, can be noticed in various ways in a clinical setting and play a decisive role in treatment. For depressive patients, these memories are usually not associated with a life-threatening situation and usually do not fulfill the criteria for posttraumatic stress disorder (PTSD), especially not Criterion A. However, they are capable of being resolved in an effective and lasting manner through EMDR therapy, as is the case for PTSD. Through this treatment, the depressive symptoms of most patients decrease with increased processing of pathogenic memories.

According to our observations, this treatment approach leads not only to a noticeably higher number of patients who completely lose their depressive symptoms at the end of treatment (complete remission), but also appears to reduce noticeably depressive relapses. In our opinion, this new therapeutic approach, developed in the course of our collective research project, can help successfully treat more patients with depressive illnesses.

A series of experiences in clinical practice have given us hope for improving the treatment of patients suffering from severe depression through this new treatment method. Consider the following patient.

Case Study I.1

TREATING AN ADULT FEMALE DIAGNOSED WITH SEVERE DEPRESSIVE EPISODE AND BORDERLINE PERSONALITY DISORDER WITH EMDR THERAPY

A 50-year-old woman was doing very poorly at the beginning of her outpatient psychotherapeutic treatment. She was severely depressed and had difficulty maintaining her daily routine. She suffered from sleep disorders, panic attacks, feelings of anxiety in several situations in life, and difficulty controlling her anger and maintaining relationships. At times, she had problems with alcohol and an eating disorder. She described intrusive memories of sexual abuse in her childhood that lasted from ages 3 to 10 without developing into PTSD. Her psychiatric case history reached as far back as she could remember and included over 10 depressive episodes, more than five hospital stays in the psychiatric ward, and three attempts at suicide. At the beginning of her treatment, she lived on welfare. The diagnosis of a severe depressive episode with repeated relapses as well as a borderline personality disorder was made.

In the first phase of the treatment, the therapist worked with classic cognitive behavioral approaches, such as questioning of irrational beliefs, the attempt to strengthen desired behaviors, as well as strategies for reducing symptoms. This was partially successful, but it did little to change her mood and depression. It did not change the patient's intrusive thoughts, which were connected with feelings of self-contempt and shame. In the middle of the therapeutic treatment, the patient heard about EMDR and asked the therapist to try it. After a few EMDR sessions to stabilize the patient, her difficult experiences were treated in eight EMDR sessions working with those memories. Two distressing experiences of separation came into focus. These experiences corresponded chronologically with the beginning of a depressive episode. Afterward, memories of the sexual assaults as well as the patient's recurring experiences of abandonment were targeted. In the course of reprocessing, the patient's self-esteem noticeably improved and at the end of the last EMDR session, she had a positive and warm feeling about her body for the first time. At the end of the 80 sessions of treatment, the patient was stable and felt markedly better. Although her depression had not completely disappeared at this point in time, she had lost her borderline personality disorder diagnosis and the majority of her borderline symptoms.

In a follow-up 6 years after the end of her treatment, she felt much better and reported she no longer had any depressive episodes. Her borderline symptoms had resolved and she had stopped all medications. Also, she had rejoined the workforce and was well enough to have responsibility for coworkers. In spite of intense, distressing experiences and more than 10 earlier depressive episodes, she could deal with more recent distressing situations well and without a depressive relapse.

Twelve years after the end of her treatment, there was another follow-up. Over this time period, she had no depressive relapses. This woman was stable and even recommended psychotherapeutic treatment to others!

Depressive disorders can present differently and run different courses. The vast literature and numerous studies on the subject are almost impossible to survey. In order to introduce our clinical approach and our manual for treating depressive disorders with EMDR (which is constantly being updated), we would like to address several fundamental situations for the treatment of depressive disorders in this introduction.

DEPRESSIVE DISORDERS

Depression is one of the most common psychological disorders. According to the research criteria of the World Health Organization's (WHO) *International Classification of Diseases, Tenth Edition (ICD-10*; WHO, 1992), depression is characterized by the following features:

1. Depressed mood, to a degree clearly unusual for the individual, most of the day, almost every day, essentially unaffected by circumstances, and persisting for at least 2 weeks
2. Interest and pleasure loss in activities that were normally enjoyable
3. Decreased drive or increased fatigue
4. Loss of self-confidence or self-esteem
5. Unfounded self-reproach or pronounced, inappropriate feelings of guilt
6. Recurrent thoughts of death or suicide, suicidal behavior
7. Complaints or evidence of decreased ability to think or concentrate, indecisiveness or indecision
8. Psychomotor agitation or inhibition
9. Sleep disturbances of any kind

10. Morning sickness
11. Loss of appetite or increased appetite with corresponding change in weight
12. Loss of libido

Exclusion criteria are:

1. The episode is not due to abuse of psychotic substances or to an organic mental disorder.
2. No manic or hypomanic symptoms are reported.

According to WHO (2017), depression affects more than 300 million people globally. The risk of developing depression (all forms) during one's lifetime is approximately 16% to 20%, internationally (Ebmeier et al., 2006). The Substance Abuse and Mental Health Services Administration (SAMHSA, 2017) estimated 17.3 million adults in the United States had at least one major depressive episode; this number represented 7.1% of all U.S. adults. The prevalence of major depressive episodes was higher among adult females (8.7%) compared to males (5.3%). The incidence of adults with a major depressive episode was highest among individuals aged 18 to 25 years (13%) and among adults reporting an ethnicity of two or more races (11.3%). Depressive episodes cause significant impairment in many people suffering from them. In 2017, an estimated 11 million U.S. adults aged 18 or older had at least one major depressive episode with severe impairment. This number represented 63.8% of all adults who reached the criteria for major depressive episodes and 4.5% of all U.S. adults.

In 2018, the Centers for Disease Control and Prevention (CDC) reported that suicide was the tenth leading cause of death in the United States, claiming the lives of over 48,000 people. Suicide was the second leading cause of death among individuals between the ages of 10 and 34, and the fourth leading cause of death among individuals between the ages of 35 and 54. Nearly all patients with severe depression have suicidal ideation. It is important to note that the number of suicide attempts are approximately 10 times higher than the number of completed suicides. For higher age groups, the number of suicide attempts—as well as the number of fatal suicide attempts—increases considerably. As one of the main risks of a depressive disorder is suicide, and since the number of cases of depression is increasing, WHO predicts that by the year 2030, unipolar depression will be the number one cause of life lost through illness (Schneider et al., 2012; WHO, 2004).

In approximately a fifth of patients who suffer from depressive episodes, hypomanic or manic episodes occur. These *bipolar disorders* are differentiated from *unipolar depression* and considered a separate illness. We will address these disorders in detail later in this text. In the following chapters, when we discuss depression, we will mostly discuss unipolar major depression.

About 60% of people with depression additionally suffer from another mental illness. The most common are anxiety disorders, addictions, and PTSD. Depressive disorders also occur frequently in conjunction with severe physical illnesses. In fact, depression is also associated by itself with a higher rate of mortality—independent of suicide. For instance, the risk of cardiovascular death is considerably higher for people suffering from depression. According to a recent investigation (Ladwig et al., 2017), the risk of depressive patients dying for a cardiovascular reason was shown to be higher than the risks that occur with hypercholesterinemia and obesity.

Many cases of depression are undiagnosed or never treated. This represents an important, stand-alone problem in the care of these people, and many efforts are currently being made to resolve this problem.

It is interesting that many depressive illnesses have "antecedents" in childhood and adolescence. These early depressive antecedents represent a discrete risk factor for depression later in life. According to Wartberg et al's (2018) representative study of 12- to 17-year-olds in Germany, 8.2% of the young people questioned were already affected by depressive symptoms. Other studies show that depressive symptoms of this kind (or depressive episodes) in adolescents represent a significant risk factor for depression later on by two to four times (Pine et al., 1998). Also, studies show that depression in childhood and adolescence are frequently connected with distressing and traumatic experiences. These young people have a significantly more complicated and difficult course of development compared with those who have depressive illnesses that develop later (Nanni et al., 2012).

Cases of depression are characterized by a progression in phases (episodes). A depressive episode is a period characterized by the symptoms of Major Depressive Disorder. In the time before psychotropic medications were introduced, the symptoms of major depression disappeared in most patients after 6 to 8 months without therapeutic interventions (Üstün et al., 2004). The development of effective therapies, like antidepressive medications and psychotherapy approaches, led to a shortening of this time to about 4 months and a less strong manifestation during individual episodes (Kessler et al., 2003). Some researchers suspect that antidepressive medications have the effect of suppressing symptoms rather than actually addressing the causes of the illness (Hollon, Thase, et al., 2002).

Depressive disorders run a course that has a great degree of variability. Both the number of depressive episodes and whether depressive symptoms have disappeared completely (complete remission) play an important role for the further development of the illness. Patients frequently experience symptoms that remain after an incomplete remission as limiting. Remaining symptoms of this kind represent one of the strongest risk factors for a depressive relapse (Nierenberg et al., 2003). It is estimated that the risk for a depressive relapse—in the case of an incomplete remission of the depressive disorder—is about five times higher than for a patient with a complete remission. On average, the expected probability of a remission 2 years after the completion of a successful treatment of a depressive disorder is 40% to 50% (de Jong-Meyer et al., 2007; Hollon et al., 1992).

Internationally, it is calculated that only 20% to 30% of depressive patients suffer from a single depressive episode. Seventy-eight percent of patients suffer from repeated episodes, depending on the length of observation (Angst, 1986; Greden, 2002). The probability of suffering from depression again increases after a second episode by 70% and by the third episode the probability is around 90% (Kupfer, 1991). When there is an accelerated occurrence of the next episode, patients are more likely to be resistant to treatment (Keller et al., 1998). For about 20% of patients, the illness becomes chronic (Eaton et al., 2008, Keller et al., 1992). For the vast majority of depressive patients, it can be assumed that the illness is either chronic or recurs in phases (the depressive episodes).

CURRENT POSSIBILITIES FOR TREATMENT AND THEIR LIMITS

Alongside watchful waiting, which is used for less severe cases of depression, there are three fundamental therapeutic approaches, as well as a series of additional established therapeutic methods for the treatment of depressive disorders. The most frequently used forms of treatment are medication, psychotherapeutic treatment, as well as a combination of medication and psychotherapeutic treatment. Additional therapeutic processes that are often used supplementally—in combination with the forms of therapy already mentioned—include: light therapy, wake therapy, sports and movement therapy, electroconvulsive therapy (ECT), and transcranial magnetic stimulation (TMS), as well as occupational therapy used in inpatient treatment, such as art therapy, and body psychotherapy (Deutschen Gesellschaft für Psychiatrie und Psychotherapie, Psychosomatik und Nervenheilkunde [DGPPN] et al., 2015). All of these therapeutic options have improved the treatment of depressive illnesses, in some cases considerably. Nonetheless, some fundamental problems in the treatment of depressive patients remain unsolved today. These unsolved problems in treatment continue to lead to a high number of severely depressed people, especially those who suffer from repeated depressive episodes or repeatedly experience only short-term relief or no relief at all from their chronic severe depression.

First, we discuss the three fundamental therapeutic approaches for the treatment of depressive disorders, which have been established in most international medical guidelines. Some of the other therapeutic processes are discussed in the remainder of the book.

Medication

The option of treating depression through medication has made providing therapy for depressive patients considerably easier. It has brought relief and hope to many patients with nearly unbearable depressive conditions. As a result, there are a large number of RCTs about the effectiveness of antidepressants. In these studies, an improvement of at least 50% in the symptoms of the patients is seen as proof for the clinically relevant efficacy of these medications. In the scientific studies on treatment through medication, generally about 50% to 60% of the patients receiving treatment for 4 to 12 weeks see an improvement or a response to the medication (Walsh et al., 2002). However, a complete disappearance of depressive symptoms, that is, a complete remission, occurs usually only for fewer than half of the patients (Bauer et al., 2005). In long-term follow-ups, it is shown that many of the patients appear to oscillate back and forth between states of partial remission, complete remission, and a recurrence of symptoms. For 15% to 20% of depressive patients, in spite of treatment their depression becomes chronic with problems persisting for over 2 years (Spijker et al., 2002).

An additional important problem is the occurrence of depressive relapses. These relapses are reduced through medication only in part, even with the continuous use of medication (maintenance therapy). If one considers the risk of remission altogether, then it is about 30% to 40% after the first year, depending on the type of treatment (Belsher & Costello, 1988). After a period of 2 years following a successful treatment, a probability of relapse of 40% to 50% must be anticipated.

Furthermore, it is increasingly clear that the perception of the public, including specialists, tends to overestimate the efficacy of antidepressants. This is in part because studies that show a higher efficacy of antidepressants are published more frequently than those in which this was not the case (Elkin et al., 1989).

It has also been shown in recent meta-analyses of clinical studies that, for mild or moderate cases of depression, the clinical effect of medication must be evaluated as a placebo effect, that is, without its own demonstrable, substance-related efficacy. In these meta-analyses (Fournier et al., 2010), a clinically significant difference is only verifiable for severe depression (with scores of over 25 on the Hamilton Scale). Munkholm et al.'s (2019) meta-analysis that included 522 studies came to the conclusion that because of possible methodological errors, it remains unclear today whether antidepressants are actually more effective than placebos. An added problem with using antidepressive medications is that their long-term use is limited by side effects, such as frequent weight gain, and compliance problems that can lead to patients secretly not taking their medications (Hirschfeld, 2003; Reid & Barbui, 2010).

Overall, psychopharmacological interventions can be necessary for severe depression. However, they have limited efficacy, especially with regard to preventing chronic depression or preventing relapses. For this reason, a combination of psychopharmacotherapy and psychotherapy is usually suggested as a standard treatment in the recommendations of various international guidelines for the treatment of severe depressive disorders (DGPPN et al., 2015; National Institute for Health and Care [NICE], 2018). In actual clinical practice, this recommended procedure is frequently not observed for various reasons.

Psychotherapy

Psychotherapeutic interventions have a long tradition in the treatment of depression. The psychotherapeutic approaches for depressive disorders that are most commonly used and have a good scientific basis include cognitive behavioral therapy (CBT), psychodynamic psychotherapy, and interpersonal psychotherapy (IPT). Many studies and meta-analyses demonstrate that these psychotherapeutic approaches for the treatment of depressive episodes are at least as effective as medication (DeRubeis et al., 2005; Hollon, Muñoz, et al., 2002). Even if one assumes that about 5% to 10% of patients treated via psychotherapy will experience a temporary worsening of their status, these side effects appear more acceptable for many patients when compared with the side effects of medication.

In comparison to a treatment only with medication, psychotherapy appears to have many advantages overall. A meta-analysis of 28 studies found that a treatment with CBT—by itself or in combination with pharmaceuticals—significantly improved the results of treatment. The risk of a relapse or a relapse at the end of maintenance therapy was also significantly reduced (Beck, 2005; Hollon et al., 2006; Vittengl et al., 2007). Hence, for the treatment of a depressive disorder, many guidelines recommend that an appropriate psychotherapeutic follow-up treatment (maintenance therapy) should be offered following acute care.

These recommendations are important also because the rates of relapse, even for patients who have had a successful psychotherapeutic treatment, are high. In a study, 29% of patients suffered a new depressive episode after 1 year and 54% suffered an episode after 2 years (Vittengl et al., 2007). Similar rates are found in a number of other studies.

Many clinicians and researchers therefore view depression increasingly as a severe chronic illness that can be cured completely only in a small number of patients (Nierenberg et al., 2003). This is one of the reasons why an increasing number of researchers are searching for new approaches to the understanding and treatment of depressive disorders (Buckman et al., 2018; Heinz et al., 2016; Kraus et al., 2019).

CONSIDERING A FACTOR AGAIN: DISTRESSING EXPERIENCES

Depressive disorders can occur in very different situations, and potential causes and triggers have been analyzed in many scientific studies. Because there does not appear to be one single cause, researchers attempt to identify the factors that can contribute to the development of depression and, when possible, to find new therapeutic approaches through this investigation. Several of the established risk factors for the occurrence of a depressive episode include: genetic factors, hormonal factors, lack of exposure to light as a result of changing of the seasons, insufficient movement, social and demographic factors, rumination, certain medications, but also earlier depressive episodes and the skin condition acne, as well as other forms of chronic inflammation (Bullmore, 2018; Vallerand et al., 2018).

Two of the most important influential variables, that have repeatedly been the subject of investigation over the many years of development of therapeutic approaches to treating depressive illnesses, are genetic factors, which researchers hoped would lead to new pharmaceutical treatment approaches, and distressing or traumatic life experiences. In the last few years, especially due to recent results in neurobiological stress and trauma research, there seems to be evidence for a stronger connection between these two causal factors as the severity of stressful or traumatic life events increases.

Researchers became aware of the contribution of genetic factors to the risk for a depressive illness early on through the fact that in 50% of cases in monozygotic twins, depressive illnesses appeared in both twins (concordance rate for dizygotic twins amounts to 15%–20%). However, the search for the single genetic factor that leads to depressive disorders has had only little success. Even as new *candidate genes* are repeatedly found as risk factors for depressive disorders, it can be assumed, for the time being, that the genetic factors contributing to depressive illnesses are caused by a complex interaction among various genes.

An example of the long discussion about candidate genes can be found in studies about the variants of the serotonin transporter gene. This gene is one of the best researched candidate genes related to the occurrence of depressive episodes. In an investigation by Avshalom Caspi, a variant of this gene (with a short allele), in conjunction with several stressful life events, showed a significant influence on an increased occurrence of depressive disorders (Caspi et al., 2003).

Six years after this study, Neil Risch, one of the leading American molecular geneticists, investigated the 26 RCT studies already addressing this question in a meta-analysis. Risch et al. (2009) concluded that the connection between the variants of the serotonin transporter gene and the occurrence of a depressive disorder could not be substantiated. Moreover, it was also not possible to establish a connection between the gene variant coupled with several distressing life experiences and the occurrence of a depressive disorder. The only significant connection that this meta-analysis could establish was the connection between distressing life experiences by themselves and the occurrence of a depressive disorder (Risch et al., 2009).

In a more recent meta-analysis, 18 additional candidate genes were investigated over a series of large samples concerning their influence on the development of depressive illnesses. Just as in the study by Risch et al., there was no connection between depression and the candidate genes alone or in conjunction with distressing environmental situations. Only distressing environmental situations showed strong effects in terms of the development of depressive disorders. The authors determined that "in agreement with the recent recommendations of the National Institute of Mental Health Council Workgroup on Genomics, we conclude that it is time for depression research to abandon historical candidate gene and candidate gene-by-environment interaction hypotheses" (Border et al., 2019, p. 386).

According to these results, it does seem to be the case that possible genetic factors take a back seat to distressing life experiences, the factor shown as much more influential in the meta-analyses. But genetic studies such as these are not the only evidence for the increasingly important factor of distressing and traumatic life experiences.

From the perspective of clinical research, distressing experiences in childhood and trauma, alongside their neurobiological consequences, are now regarded as a significant factor in the causation and development of depressive episodes (Heim & Nemeroff, 2001; Nanni et al., 2012). In their investigations, Martin Teicher and his team (2006) at McLean Hospital in Boston were able to confirm not only the relationship of mistreatment and sexual abuse in early childhood with a higher risk for depression, but also the relationship of depression with emotional and verbal abuse and neglect, that is to some extent even stronger (Khan et al., 2015). In further investigations, clear neurological changes could be identified, that are caused by stressors of these kinds at various developmental ages for boys and girls (Teicher et al., 2018).

In larger epidemiological studies, it has been shown that traumatic experiences and a dysfunctional home environment in childhood appear to be responsible for a large portion of the population-dependent risk for major depression and suicide (Dube et al., 2001, 2003).

The stressors that are associated with depressive disorders do not only encompass those *traumatic experiences* that are individually defined in the diagnostic manuals. These manuals describe such *traumatic experiences* in the context of mortal danger and can easily be differentiated in Criterion A in the current diagnostic manuals of WHO or the American Psychiatric Association (APA). Important stressors that are considered clear risk factors for depression later in life are not accounted for in Criterion A; however, they are frequently accounted for concerning *attachment traumas*. This is especially the case for separations and losses, but it also applies to neglect and emotional abuse, which have a proven connection to depressive episodes. It is interesting to note that the neurobiological consequences of childhood attachment traumas of these kinds have a similar severity to the consequences of physical violence. Distressing attachment and relationship experiences appear to be much more substantial risk factors for later depressive disorders than has been previously thought (Chapman et al., 2004; Minelli et al., 2019; Teicher et al., 2006). Studies of depressive patients have additionally shown that they, in comparison to healthy control persons, have suffered from two to three times as many experiences of loss early in life (Agid et al., 1999).

Distressing experiences that are associated with a risk for depression or with a direct trigger for a depressive episode do not only occur in childhood. Studies have also shown that experiences of separation, loss, embarrassment, and humiliation, even in adulthood, have a clearly demonstrable connection to the beginning of depressive episodes. Even bullying or chronic psychosocial stress at work significantly increases the risk for depression (Siegrist, 2008). In clinical interviews, many depressive patients can even name the situations and circumstances that they associate with the beginning of their depressive illness. Perhaps it is a good thing that research increasingly suggests we should dedicate more attention to the distressing experiences patients describe in these contexts, even if these experiences do not satisfy the criteria of a traumatic trigger situation (Criterion A).

At this point, the concept of trauma as an attachment trauma in connection with depression, which was already described in the classical psychoanalytic literature, is becoming more important (Bowlby, 1980; Brisch, 2017; Wöller, 2006). The classic concept of trauma, that is limited to distressing experiences that fulfill Criterion A, appears admittedly to be helpful in the context of PTSD, but seems to fall short for distressing experiences that appear in the context of depressive disorders. The question here is, in fact, whether experiences of this kind that appear to be illness triggering and pathogenic, but do not fulfill Criterion A for PTSD, should all be described under the term *trauma,* which is narrowly defined in the diagnostic manuals.

Another way to account for these distressing experiences, which are at times difficult to classify, is to return to the nine adverse childhood experiences that are part of the *Adverse Childhood Experiences* (*ACEs*) studies. ACEs are not limited to classic trauma in childhood; they also incorporate many influences from the household and social environment of the child. During an interview, it is possible to ask patients if they have experienced any of the ACEs by simply responding *yes* or *no*. (In more recent ACEs studies, particular forms of distressing experiences have been added or left out; however, the results remain fundamentally the same.) The classic ACE list contains the following nine risk factors:

- Repeated physical abuse
- Repeated emotional abuse
- Sexual abuse with physical contact
- Alcoholic or drug addict in the household
- Member of the household in prison
- Member of the household with chronic depression, mental illness, in inpatient treatment, or suicidal
- Single parent or no parents
- Emotional or mental neglect

Every *yes* to a question from the list counted for one point.

The first ACEs study arose from a cooperative effort between the CDC and the department of preventive medicine for a major American insurance company in San Diego, California. In the study, over 17,000 middle-class Americans (average age: 57 years old) were surveyed using the ACE list, while they also answered questions about their health and illnesses. The results showed a highly significant correlation between the ACE point values (0–9 points were possible in total) and mental health problems like depression, suicide attempts, and substance abuse. For patients with depressive illnesses, they found that these depressive symptoms were more difficult to treat in adulthood when there were also more severe stress factors in childhood, especially physical abuse and neglect (Infurna et al., 2016; Nanni et al., 2012).

Furthermore, there were strong connections between ACE factors and risk behaviors such as smoking or teenage pregnancy, a heightened risk of traumatization and of perpetrating abuse oneself, as well as a correlation with a number of severe physical illnesses such as hypertension, coronary heart disease and heart attack, lung disease, and/or HIV (Anda et al., 2006; Felitti et al., 1998). This study has been repeated many times internationally and its results have been confirmed in a meta-analysis by Professor Karin Hughes of the European Regional Office of WHO, who provided a new analysis of 37 of these studies, encompassing over 250,000 participants (Hughes et al., 2017).

It is interesting to note that the ACEs studies show a clear, cumulative dose-response effect in the number of kinds of distressing experiences and depressive symptoms—a higher degree of distress also leads to stronger symptoms (Witt et al., 2019a, 2019b). This dose-response relationship is also shown in other studies about depressive disorders (Mollica et al., 1998; Shore et al., 1986a, 1986b; Wise et al., 2001) and is illustrated in Figure I.1. There are other studies that have shown a temporal connection between distressing experiences and the occurrence of depressive symptoms. This temporal connection was markedly closer for depression than what was shown for anxiety disorders and events with mortal danger (Kendler & Gardner, 2016; Kendler et al., 2003; Strauss et al., 2018). Both correlations, the temporal connection of event and falling ill, as well as the dose-response relationship, suggest a causal relationship between distressing or traumatic experiences and the occurrence of depressive episodes.

The correlation between severe distressing experiences, which can only be partially accounted for in WHO's definition for *traumatic* life experiences, and depressive disorders has by now been well established by scientific studies and has been discussed for over 10 years in the literature. However, these results have hardly had any impact on the actual treatment of depressive patients.

In our clinical experience and practice, we have developed and used new approaches to trauma-centered psychotherapy. We have found increasing evidence and practical examples for the success of a new therapeutic approach for depressive disorders. This method is EMDR therapy. In this new therapeutic approach, based on trauma-centered psychotherapy, the traumatic memories as well as the distressing ones and their consequences can be directly brought into focus and processed.

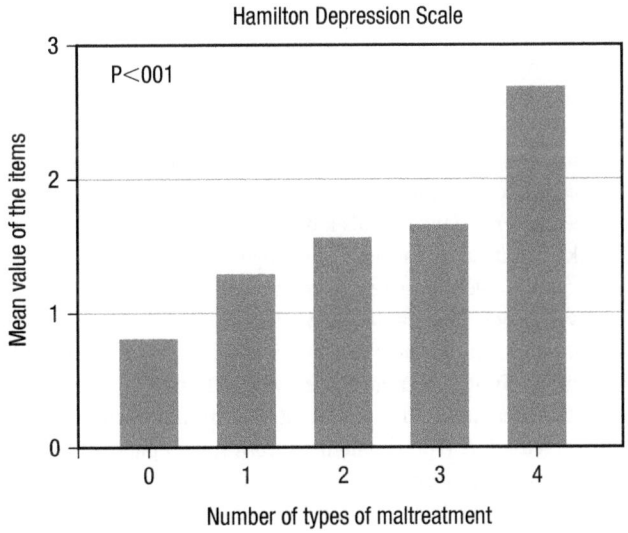

FIGURE I.1 Dose-response relationship between the number of forms of abuse and depressive symptoms as seen in the Hamilton Depression Rating Scale.

Source: Data from Khan, A., McCormack, H. C., Bolger, E. A., McGreenery, C. E., Vitaliano, G., Polcari, A., & Teicher, M. H. (2015). Childhood maltreatment, depression, and suicidal ideation: Critical importance of parental and peer emotional abuse during developmental sensitive periods in males and females. *Frontiers in Psychiatry*, 6, 42. https://doi.org/10.3389/fpsyt.2015.00042

PATHOGENIC MEMORIES AND EMDR THERAPY

The basis of this new approach is the model of pathogenic memories that develop as memory networks after classic traumatic events and also after non-traumatic, distressing experiences such as separations and losses, and in other situations, in response to pain or addictive substances (Hase et al., 2017). The model for pathogenic memories builds on Francine Shapiro's Adaptive Information Processing (AIP) Model, postulated in 2001, that already pointed to the special way in which distressing experiences are stored and remembered (dysfunctionally stored memories). Pathogenic memories are biologically active, single memories, or complexes of memories that are usually associated with autonomic vegetative activation and symptoms linked with this disturbance (like arousal or intrusions of memory fragments).

Patients can usually judge and rate the *disturbance* of these memories very well. Shapiro uses this fact by modifying Joseph Wolpe's Subjective Units of Disturbance (SUD) scale and integrating it into EMDR therapy (Shapiro, 1995; Wolpe, 1969). Patients can use the resulting 11-point Likert scale to rate the degree of their subjective distress from 0 to 10. Patients are asked: *On a scale from 0–10, where 0 means no disturbance or neutral and 10 is the highest disturbance you can imagine, how disturbing does the memory feel to you now?* This scale can be used very well in treatment, has good psychometric characteristics, and is a helpful indicator for therapeutic changes in EMDR therapy (Kim et al., 2008). The decrease of SUD in EMDR therapy is significantly correlated with a decrease in autonomic vegetative symptoms (Sack et al., 2008). In an investigation using electroencephalography (EEG), Pagani et al. (2012) showed that with PTSD patients, the neuronal activity in the brain was strongly centered in the limbic, and subcortical area during the activation of a pathogenic memory. After successful EMDR treatment, the neuronal activity had shifted to the associative cortical area during the activation of the memory and was no longer experienced as distressing.

Most depressive patients who can associate a triggering experience with the beginning of their depressive episode give a high value on the SUD scale when asked about this experience. This occurs frequently even when these distressing experiences (losses, separation, bullying, etc.) have already been processed (discussed) in psychotherapy. For many of these patients, the time interval between an experience of this kind and the beginning of the depressive episode is about 4 to 8 weeks, but it can occasionally be longer. Even when the connections for some patients are more complex, we call these events *Episode Trigger(s)* as they relate to the beginning of the depressive episode. One way to test whether patients with a depressive episode could profit from EMDR therapy is to ask them about their current level of distress (SUD) with regard to the suspected Episode Trigger. In many cases, you will find that, even for experiences that have already been discussed and understood multiple times in treatment, the level of distress remains markedly increased. A typical statement from such a patient would be, *I understand the event much better today and can also deal with it better. But it still feels very distressing for me.*

It appears that, there has been some improvement in the cortical/cognitive understanding of their depressive problems, but the distress can still be felt due to the pathogenic memories that are overwhelmingly entrenched in the limbic area. Frequently, after successful psychotherapeutic treatment, residual symptoms remain that not only hinder the complete disappearance of symptoms but also can increase the risk of depressive relapses later on.

FIRST SYSTEMATIC INVESTIGATIONS

Our first systematic study, designed to test the efficacy of using EMDR therapy for depressive patients in this way, was a retrospective study we began in 2008. We had already heard from a number of colleagues who were reporting on depressive disorders treated successfully with EMDR. Some also reported that patients who had previously always relapsed into depressive episodes had their relapses end after an EMDR treatment.

We wanted to investigate this more systematically. The EMDR-Institut Deutschland (EMDR Institute of Germany), founded in 1992, is an institute for education and research that has a network of lecturers and supervisors across Germany at its disposal. In this network, we asked experienced trainers of EMDR if they had treated patients with recurring depression PTSD using EMDR therapy. Here, we were particularly interested in treatments that ended successfully and took place some time ago. We then asked our colleagues to contact these patients again and to find out how they were doing concerning their depressive symptoms. Here, we were particularly interested in relapses that had occurred in the meantime. Patients were additionally asked to fill out a Beck Depression Inventory once again.

In total, we were able to find 10 patients (nine women, one man) for this study. The average age was 52 years old, all had recurring depression (*ICD-10*: F33.X), and two had so-called double depression (*ICD-10*: F33.X and F34.1). For three patients, the depression had already become chronic and had persisted for over 2 years. The average number of relapses was equal to 6.4, with a range of three to 13. All of the patients had been in out-patient psychotherapeutic treatment using CBT or psychodynamic therapy. The length of treatment amounted to 60 sessions on average, out of which pathogenic memories had been processed with EMDR therapy in 7.4 sessions. Only one patient had received 10 treatment sessions where pathogenic memories were processed with EMDR in four sessions. The follow-ups occurred on average 3.7 years after the end of treatment (range of 1–6 years). We knew from the patients' records that 70% of them had reached a complete remission of their depressive symptoms after the end of therapy.

In the follow-up, it was shown that by this point in time, 90% reported a full remission of their depressive symptoms. This was confirmed through the questionnaires they returned (Beck Depression Inventory, Second Edition [BDI-II]). Only the patient who received 10 therapy sessions (four of which were EMDR sessions) reported two short depressive episodes, which passed after a 3-month treatment with antidepressants. The trigger for these episodes had been her husband falling severely ill. Only one other patient, who during her depressive episode had shortly had psychotic symptoms, reported at the time of the follow-up that she was still taking medication. The rest of her cohort no longer required medication. It was interesting to note that three of the patients reported severely distressing experiences since the end of their treatment. However, these did not lead to a depressive episode (one suffered a heart attack, another's spouse died, and another's house caught fire). It seemed as if the patients' resilience had increased since their treatment.

Altogether, these results, especially the *lack* of depressive relapses, were very impressive to us, especially as we knew that the high number of relapses for depressive disorders was an important clinical problem. For the first time, we saw the possibility, as a result of this case series, to change the trajectory for many depressive patients by means of EMDR therapy. Although we were unable to publish this study at the time, it was decisively encouraging and motivated us to pursue further systematic investigations about the use of EMDR in the treatment of depression.

In 2010, these findings led to the founding of the international European Depression EMDR Network (EDEN) working group. Currently, our group has published five controlled studies, including three RCT studies, about the use of EMDR therapy for depressive disorders.

In total, nine RCT studies have been published about EMDR in the treatment of depression at the time of this book's publication (a list of these RCT studies can be found in Chapter 13 of this book). These studies show that EMDR therapy is at least comparable to conventional forms of treatment and give indications that this method may give a stronger resolution of depressive symptoms of this hard-to-treat population (Malandrone et al., 2019).

The research we have begun since these first investigations and pursued through these controlled studies have led our working group to a number of conclusions about the possibility of using EMDR therapy for patients successfully in the clinical setting. We would like to present these conclusions in this book. These strategies have been developed from the results of our controlled studies and the outpatient and inpatient treatment of over 500 patients with depressive disorders. A central element of this is represented by our structured strategy, that we have put into a manual (Hofmann et al., 2016). The chapters in Part II of this book correspond to the structure of this manual (EMDR DeprEnd manual).

In this book, there are also suggestions on how to find a good EMDR therapist (Chapter 15), as well as an EMDR drawing protocol (Chapter 9) representing an additional option for treatment that dovetails well with EMDR therapy. You also will find a list of all RCT studies on EMDR and depression (Chapter 13) and instructions on how to use the Symptom Event Map (Chapter 14).

Although many questions remain open and although EMDR therapy is not the best treatment option for all patients, we believe that our approach can provide helpful strategies for the treatment of many depressive patients.

REFERENCES

Agid, O., Shapira, B., Zislin, J., Ritsner, M., Hanin, B., Murad, H., Troudart, T., Bloch, M., Heresco-Levy, U., & Lerer, B. (1999). Environment and vulnerability to major psychiatric illness: A case control study of early parental loss in major depression, bipolar disorder and schizophrenia. *Molecular Psychiatry, 4*(2), 163–172. https://doi.org/10.1038/sj.mp.4000473

Anda, R. F., Felitti, V. J., Bremner, J. D., Walker, J. D., Whitfield, C. L., Perry, B. D., Dube, S. R., & Giles, W. H. (2006). The enduring effects of abuse and related adverse experiences in childhood. A convergence of evidence from neurobiology and epidemiology. *European Archives of Psychiatry and Clinical Neuroscience, 256*(3), 174–186. https://doi.org/10.1007/s00406-005-0624-4

Angst, J. (1986). The course of affective disorders. *Psychopathology, 19*(2), 47–52. https://doi.org/10.1159/000285131

Bauer, M., Berghöfer, A., & Adli, M. (2005). *Akute und therapieresistente Depressionen: Pharmakotherapie – psychotherapie – innovationen* (2. Aufl.). Springer Medizin Verlag.

Beck, A. T. (2005). The current state of cognitive therapy: A 40-year retrospective. *Archives of General Psychiatry, 62*(9), 953–959. https://doi.org/10.1001/archpsyc.62.9.953

Belsher, G., & Costello, C. G. (1988). Relapse after recovery from unipolar depression: A critical review. *Psychological Bulletin Journal, 104*(1), 84–96. https://doi.org/10.1037/0033-2909.104.1.84

Border, R., Johnson, E. J., Evans, L. M., Smolen, A., Berley, N., Sullivan, P. F., & Keller, M. C. (2019). No support for historical candidate gene or candidate gene-by-interaction hypo-theses for major depression across multiple large samples. *American Journal of Psychiatry, 176*(5), 376–387. https://doi.org/10.1176/appi.ajp.2018.18070881

Bowlby, J. (1980). *Attachment and loss. Vol. III: Loss: Sadness and depression.* Basic Books.

Brisch, K. H. (2017). *Bindungstraumatisierungen.* Klett-Cotta.

Buckman, J. E. J., Underwood, A., Clarke, K., Saunders, R., Hollon, S., Fearon, P., & Pilling, S. (2018). Risk factors for relapse and recurrence of depression in adults and how they operate: A four-phase systematic review and meta-synthesis. *Clinical Psychology Review, 64*, 13–38. https://doi.org/10.1016/j.cpr.2018.07.005

Bullmore, E. (2018). The art of medicine: Inflamed depression. *The Lancet, 6*(10154), 1189–1190. https://doi.org/10.1016/S0140-6736(18)32356-0

Caspi, A., Sugden, K., Moffitt, T. E., Taylor, A., Craig, I. W., Harrington, H., McClay, J., Mill, J., Martin, J., Braithwaite, A., & Poulton, R. (2003). Influence of life stress on depression: Moderation by a polymorphism in the 5-HTT gene. *Science, 301*(5631), 386–389. https://doi.org/10.1126/science.1083968

Chapman, D. P., Whitfield, C. L., Felitti, V. J., Dube, S. R., Edwards, V. J., & Anda, R. F. (2004). Adverse childhood experiences and the risk of depressive disorders in adulthood. *Journal of Affective Disorders, 82*(2), 217–225. https://doi.org/10.1016/j.jad.2003.12.013

de Jong-Meyer, R., Hautzinger, M., Kühner, C., & Schramm, E. (2007). *Evidenzbasierte Leitlinien zur Psychotherapie Affektiver Störungen*. Hogrefe.

DeRubeis, R. J., Hollon, S. D., Amsterdam, J. D., Shelton, R. C., Young, P. R., Salomon, R. M., O'Reardon, J. P., Lovett, M. L., Gladis, M. M., Brown, L. L., & Gallop, R. (2005). Cognitive therapy vs medications in the treatment of moderate to severe depression. *Archives of General Psychiatry, 62*(4), 409–416. https://doi.org/10.1001/archpsyc.62.4.409

Deutschen Gesellschaft für Psychiatrie und Psychotherapie, Psychosomatik und Nerven-heilkunde, Bundesärztekammer, Kassenärztliche Bundesvereinigung, Arbeitsgemeinschaft wissenschaftlicher Medizinischer Fachgesellschaften. (Eds.). (2015). *S3-Leitlinie/Nationale Versorgungsleitlinie Unipolare Depression (German National Guideline on Unipolar Depression)* (2nd ed.; Version 5). https://doi.org/10.6101/AZQ/000364; www.depression.versorgungsleitlinien.de

Dube, S. R., Anda, R. F., Felitti, V. J., Chapman, D., Williamson, D. F., & Giles, W. H. (2001). Childhood abuse, household dysfunction, and the risk of attempted suicide throughout the life span: Findings from the Adverse Childhood Experiences Study. *Journal of the American Medical Association, 286*(24), 3089–3096. https://doi.org/10.1001/jama.286.24.3089

Dube, S. R., Felitti, V. J., Dong, M., Chapman, D. P., Giles, W. H., & Anda, R. F. (2003). Childhood abuse, neglect, and household dysfunction and the risk of illicit drug use: The Adverse Childhood Experiences Study. *Pediatrics, 111*(3), 564–572. https://doi.org/10.1542/peds.111.3.564

Eaton, W. W., Shao, H., Nestadt, G., Lee, B. H., Bienvenu, O. J., & Zandi, P. (2008). Population-based study of first onset and chronicity in major depressive disorder. *Archives of General Psychiatry, 65*(5), 513–520. https://doi.org/10.1001/archpsyc.65.5.513

Ebmeier, K. P., Donaghey, C., & Steele, J. D. (2006). Recent developments and current controversies in depression. *The Lancet, 267*, 153–167. https://doi.org/10.1016/S0140-6736(06)67964-6

Elkin, I., Shea, M. T., Watkins, J. T., Imber, S. D., Sotsky, S. M., Collins, J. F., Glass, D. R., Pilkonis, P. A., Leber, W. R., Docherty, J. P., Fiester, S. J., & Parloff, M. B. (1989). National Institute of Mental Health Treatment of Depression Collaborative Research Program: General effectiveness of treatments. *Archives of General Psychiatry, 46*(11), 971–982. https://doi.org/10.1001/archpsyc.1989.01810110013002

Felitti, V. J., Anda, R. F., Nordenberg, D., Williamson, D. F., Spitz, A. M., Edwards, V., Koss, M. P., & Marks, J. S. (1998). Relationship of childhood abuse and household dysfunction to many of the leading causes of death in adults. The Adverse Childhood Experience (ACE) Study. *American Journal of Preventive Medicine, 14*(4), 245–258. https://doi.org/10.1016/s0749-3797(98)00017-8

Fournier, J. C., DeRubeis, R. J., Hollon, S. D., Dimidjian, S., Amsterdam, J. D., Shelton, R. C., & Fawcett, J. (2010). Antidepressant drug effects and depression severity: A patient-level meta-analysis. *Journal of the American Association, 303*(1), 47–53. https://doi.org/10.1001/jama.2009.1943

Greden, J. F. (2002). Unmet need: What justifies the search for a new antidepressant? *Journal of Clinical Psychiatry, 63*(Suppl 2), 3–7. PMID: 15453007.

Hase, M., Balmaceda, U. M., Hase, A., Lehnung, M., Tumani, V., Huchzermeier, C., & Hofmann, A. (2015). Eye movement desensitization and reprocessing (EMDR) therapy in the treatment of depression: A matched pairs study in an inpatient setting. *Brain and Behavior, 5*, e00342. https://doi.org/10.1002/brb3.342

Hase, M., Balmaceda, U. M., Ostacoli, L., Liebermann, P., & Hofmann, A. (2017). The AIP model of EMDR therapy and pathogenic memories. *Frontiers in Psychology, 8*, 1578. https://doi.org/10.3389/fpsyg.2017.01578

Hase, M., Plagge, J., Hase, A., Braas, R., Ostacoli, L., Hofmann, A., & Huchzermeier, C. (2018). Eye movement desensitization and reprocessing versus treatment as usual in the treatment of depression: A randomized-controlled trial. *Frontiers in Psychology, 14*(9), 1384. https://doi.org/10.3389/fpsyg.2018.01384

Heim, C., & Nemeroff, C. B. (2001). The role of childhood trauma in the neurobiology of mood and anxiety disorders: Preclinical and clinical studies. *Biological Psychiatry, 49*(12), 1023–1039. https://doi.org/10.1016/s0006-3223(01)01157-x

Heinz, A., Schlagenhauf, F., Beck, A., & Wackerhagen, C. (2016). Dimensional psychiatry: Mental disorders as dysfunctions of basic learning mechanisms. *Journal of Neural Transmission, 123*, 809–821. https://doi.org/10.1007/s00702-016-1561-2

Hirschfeld, R. M. A. (2003). Long-term side effects of SSRIs: Sexual dysfunction and weight gain. *Journal of Clinical Psychiatry, 64*(Suppl 18), 20–24. PMID: 14700451.

Hofmann, A., Hase, M., Liebermann, P., Ostacoli, L., Lehnung, M., Ebner, F., Rost, C., Luber, M., & Tumani, V. (2016). DeprEnd® – EMDR therapy protocol for the treatment of depressive disorders. In M. Luber (Ed.), *EMDR therapy-scripted protocols and summary sheets: Treating anxiety, obsessive-compulsive, and mood-related conditions* (pp. 289–323). Springer Publishing Company.

Hollon, S. D., DeRubeis, R. J., Evans, M. D., Wiemer, M. J., Garvey, M. J., Grove, W. M., & Tuason, V. B. (1992). Cognitive therapy and pharmacotherapy for depression: Singly and in combination. *Archives of General Psychiatry, 49*(10), 774–781. https://doi.org/10.1001/archpsyc.1992.01820100018004

Hollon, S. D., Muñoz, R. F., Barlow, D. H., Beardslee, W. R., Bell, C. C., Bernal, G., Clarke, G. N., Franciosi, L. P., Kazdin, A. L., Kohn, L., Linehan, M. M., Markowitz, J. C., Miklowitz, D. J., Persons, J. B., Niederehe, G., & Sommers, D. (2002). Psychosocial intervention development for the prevention and treatment of depression: Promoting innovation and increasing access. *Biological Psychiatry, 52*(6), 610–630. https://doi.org/10.1016/s0006-3223(02)01384-7

Hollon, S. D., Steward, M. O., & Strunk, D. (2006). Enduring effects for cognitive behavior therapy in the treatment of depression and anxiety. *Annual Review of Psychology, 57*, 285–315. https://doi.org/10.1146/annurev.psych.57.102904.190044

Hollon, S. D., Thase, M. E. & Markowitz, J. C. (2002). Treatment and prevention of depression. *Psychological Science in the Public Interest, 3*(20), 39–77. https://doi.org/10.1111/1529-1006.00008

Hughes, K., Bellis, M. A., Hardcastle, K. A., Sethi, D., Butchart, A., Mikton, C., Jones, L., & Dunne, M. P. (2017). The effect of multiple adverse childhood experiences on health: A systematic review and meta-analysis. *Lancet Public Health, 2*(8), e356–e366. https://doi.org/10.1016/S2468-2667(17)30118-4

Infurna, M. R., Reichl, C., Parzer, P., Schimmenti, A., Bifulco, A., & Kaess, M. (2016). Associations between depression and specific childhood experiences of abuse and neglect: A meta-analysis. *Journal of Affective Disorders, 190*, 47–55. https://doi.org/10.1016/j.jad.2015.09.006

Keller, M. B., & Boland, R. J. (1998). Implications of failing to achieve successful long-term maintenance treatment of recurrent unipolar major depression. *Biological Psychiatry, 44*(5), 348–360. https://doi.org/10.1016/s0006-3223(98)00110-3

Keller, M. B., Lavori, P. W., Mueller, T. I., Endicott, J., Coryell, W., Hirschfeld, R. M., & Shea, T. (1992, October). Time to recovery, chronicity, and levels of psychopathology in major depression. A 5-year prospective follow-up of 431 subjects. *Archives of General Psychiatry, 49*(10), 809–816. https://doi.org/10.1001/archpsyc.1992.01820100053010

Kendler, K. S., Hettema, J. M., Butera, F., Gardner, C. O., & Prescott, C. A. (2003). Life event dimensions of loss, humiliation, entrapment, and danger in the prediction of onsets of major depression and generalized anxiety. *Archives of General Psychiatry, 60*(8), 789–796. https://doi.org/10.1001/archpsyc.60.8.789

Kendler, K. S., & Gardner, C. O. (2016). Depressive vulnerability, stressful life events and episode onset of major depression: A longitudinal model. *Psychological Medicine, 46*(9), 1865–1874. https://doi.org/10.1017/S0033291716000349

Kessler, R. C., Berglund, P., Demler, O., Jin, R., Koretz, D., Merikangas, K. R., Rush, A. J., Walters, E. E., & Wang, P. S. (2003). The epidemiology of major depressive disorder: Results from the National Comorbidity Survey Replication (NCS-R). *JAMA, 289*(23), 3095–3105. https://doi.org/10.1001/jama.289.23.3095

Khan, A., McCormack, H. C., Bolger, E. A., McGreenery, C. E., Vitaliano, G., Polcari, A., & Teicher, M. H. (2015). Childhood maltreatment, depression, and suicidal ideation: Critical importance of parental and peer emotional abuse during developmental sensitive periods in males and females. *Frontiers in Psychiatry, 6*, 42. https://doi.org/10.3389/fpsyt.2015.00042

Kim, D., Bae, H., & Yong, C. P. (2008). Validity of the Subjective Units of Disturbance Scale in EMDR. *Journal of EMDR Practice and Research, 2*(1), 57–62. https://doi.org/10.1891/1933-3196.2.1.57

Kraus, C., Kadriu, B., Lanzenberger, R., Zarate, C. A. J., & Kasper, S. (2019). Prognosis and improved outcomes in major depression: A review. *Translational Psychiatry, 9*(1), 127. https://doi.org/10.1038/s41398-019-0460-3

Kupfer, D. J. (1991). Long-term treatment of depression. *Journal of Clinical Psychiatry, 52*(Suppl), 28–34. PMID: 1903134.

Ladwig, K.-H., Baumert, J., Marten-Mittag, B., Lukaschek, K., Johar, H., Fang, X., Ronel, J., Meisinger, C., Peters, A., & KORA Investigators. (2017). Room for depressed and exhausted mood as a risk predictor for all-cause and cardiovascular mortality beyond the contribution of the classical somatic risk factors in men. *Atherosclerosis, 257*, 224–231. https://doi.org/10.1016/j.atherosclerosis.2016.12.003

Malandrone, F., Carletto, S., Hase, M., Hofmann, A., & Ostacoli, L. (2019). A brief narrative summary of randomized controlled trials investigating EMDR treatment of patients with depression. *Journal of EMDR Practice and Research, 13*(4), 302–306. https://doi.org/10.1891/1933-3196.13.4.302

Minelli, A., Zampieri, E., Sacco, C., Bazzanella, R., Mezzetti, N., Tessari, E., Barlati, S., & Bortolomasi, M. (2019). Clinical efficacy of trauma-focused psychotherapies in treatment-resistant depression (TRD) in-patients: A randomized controlled pilot-study. *Psychiatry Research, 273*, 567–574. https://doi.org/10.1016/j.psychres.2019.01.070

Mollica, R. F., McInnes, K., Poole, C., & Tor, S. (1998). Dose-effect relationships of trauma to symptoms of depression and post-traumatic stress disorder among Cambodian survivors of mass violence. *British Journal of Psychiatry, 173*(6), 482–488. https://doi.org/10.1192/bjp.173.6.482

Munkholm, K., Paludan-Müller, A. S., & Boesen, K. (2019). Considering the methodological limitations in the evidence base of antidepressants for depression: A reanalysis of a network meta-analysis. *BMJ Open, 9*, e024886. https://doi.org/10.1136/bmjopen-2018-024886

Nanni, V., Uher, R., & Danese, A. (2012). Childhood maltreatment predicts unfavorable course of illness and treatment outcome in depression: A meta-analysis. *American Journal of Psychiatry, 169*(2), 141–151. https://doi.org/10.1176/appi.ajp.2011.11020335

National Institute for Health and Care Excellence (NICE). (2018). *Clinical guideline – Depression in adults: Recognition and management.* National Institute for Health and Care Excellence.

Nierenberg, A. A., Petersen, T. J., & Alpert, J. E. (2003). Prevention of relapse and recurrence in depression: The role of long-term pharmacotherapy and psychotherapy. *Journal of Clinical Psychiatr, 64*(Suppl 15), 13–17. PMID: 14658986.

Ostacoli, L., Carletto, S., Cavallo, M., Baldomir-Gago, P., Di Lorenzo, G., Fernandez, I., Hase, M., Justo-Alonso, A., Lehnung, M., Migliaretti, G., Oliva, F., Pagani, M., Recarey-Eiris, S., Torta, R., Tumani, V., Gonzalez-Vazquez, A. I., & Hofmann, A. (2018). Comparison of eye movement desensitization reprocessing and cognitive behavioral therapy as adjunctive treatments for recurrent depression: The European Depression EMDR Network (EDEN) randomized controlled trial. *Frontiers in Psychology, 9*, Article 74. https://doi.org/10.3389/fpsyg.2018.00074

Pagani, M., Di Lorenzo, G., Verardo, A. R., Nicolais, G., Monaco, L., Lauretti, G., Russo, R., Niolu, C., Ammaniti, M., Fernandez, I., & Siracusano, A. (2012). Neurobiological correlates of EMDR monitoring – An EEG study. *PLoS ONE, 7*(9), e45753. https://doi.org/10.1371/journal.pone.0045753

Pine, D. S., Cohen, P., Gurley, D., Brook, J., & Ma, Y. (1998). The risk for early-adulthood anxiety and depressive disorders in adolescents with anxiety and depressive disorders. *Archives of General Psychiatry, 55*(1), 56–64. https://doi.org/10.1001/archpsyc.55.1.56

Reid, S., & Barbui, C. (2010). Long term treatment of depression with selective serotonin reuptake inhibitors and newer antidepressants. *British Medical Journal, 340*, 752–756. https://doi.org/10.1136/bmj.c1468

Risch, N., Herrell, R., Lehner, T., Liang, K. Y., Eaves, L., Hoh, J., Griem, A., Kovacs, M., Ott, J., & Merikangas, K. R. (2009). Interaction between the serotonin transporter gene (5-HTTLPR), stressful life events, and risk of depression. A meta-analysis. *JAMA, 301*(23), 2462–2471. https://doi.org/10.1001/jama.2009.878

Sack, M., Lempa, W., Steinmetz, A., Lamprecht, F., & Hofmann, A. (2008). Alterations in autonomic tone during trauma exposure using eye movement desensitization and reprocessing (EMDR) – Results of a preliminary investigation. *Journal of Anxiety Disorders, 22*(7), 1264–1271. https://doi.org/10.1016/j.janxdis.2008.01.007

Schneider, F., Falkai, P., & Maier, W. (2012). *Psychiatrie 2020 plus.* Springer Nature.

Shapiro, F. (1995). *Eye movement desensitization and reprocessing: Basic principles, protocols and procedures* (1st ed.). Guilford Press.

Shore, J. H., Tatum, E. L., & Vollmer, W. M. (1986a). Evaluation of mental effects of disaster, Mount St. Helens eruption. *American Journal of Public Health, 76*, 76–83. https://doi.org/10.2105/ajph.76.suppl.76

Shore, J. H., Tatum, E. L., & Vollmer, W. M. (1986b). Psychiatric reactions to disaster: The Mount St. Helens experience. *American Journal of Public Health, 143*(5), 590–595. https://doi.org/10.1176/ajp.143.5.590

Siegrist, J. (2008). Chronic psychosocial stress at work and risk of depression: Evidence from prospective studies. *European Archives of Psychiatry and Clinical Neuroscience, 258*(5), 115–119. https://doi.org/10.1007/s00406-008-5024-0

Spijker, J., de Graaf, R., Bijl, R. V., Beekman, A. T. F., Ormel, J., & Nolen, W. A. (2002). Duration of major depressive episodes in the general population: Results from the Netherlands Mental Health Survey an Incidence Study (NEMESIS). *British Journal of Psychiatry, 181*(3), 208–213. https://doi.org/10.1192/bjp.181.3.208

Strauss, M., Mergl, R., Gürke, N., Kleinert, K., Sander, C., & Hegerl, U. (2018). Association between acute critical life events and the speed of onset of depressive episodes in male and female depressed patients. *BMC Psychiatry, 18*(1), 332. https://doi.org/10.1186/s12888-018-1923-4

Substance Abuse and Mental Health Services Administration. (2017). *Major depression.* Center for Behavioral Health Statistics and Quality, National Survey on Drug Use and Health, 2016 and 2017. https://www.nimh.nih.gov/health/statistics/major-depression

Teicher, M. H., Samson, J. A., Polcari, A., & McGreenery, C. E. (2006). Sticks, stones, and hurtful words: Relative effects of various forms of childhood maltreatment. *American Journal of Psychiatry, 163*(6), 993–1000. https://doi.org/10.1176/ajp.2006.163.6.993

Teicher, M. H., Anderson, C. M., Ohashi, K., Khan, A., McGreenery, C. E., Bolger, E. A., Rohan, M. L., & Vitaliano, G. D. (2018). Differential effects of childhood neglect and abuse during sensitive exposure periods on male and female hippocampus. *NeuroImage, 169*, 443–452. https://doi.org/10.1016/j.neuroimage.2017.12.055

Üstün, T. B., Ayuso-Mateos, J. L., Chatterji, S., Mathers, C., & Murray, C. J. L. (2004). Global burden of depressive disorders in the year 2000. *British Journal of Psychiatry, 184*(5), 386–392. https://doi.org/10.1192/bjp.184.5.386

Vallerand, I. A., Lewinson, R. T., Parsons, L. M., Lowerison, M. W., Frolkis, A. D., Kaplan, G. G., Barnabe, C., Bulloch, A. G. M. & Patten, S. B. (2018). Risk of depression among patients with acne in the U.K.: A population-based cohort study. *British Journal of Dermatology, 178*(3), e194–e195. https://doi.org/10.1111/bjd.16099

Vittengl, J. R., Clark, L. A., Dunn, T. W., & Jarrett, R. B. (2007). Reducing relapse and recurrence in unipolar depression: A comparative meta-analysis of cognitive-behavioral therapy's effects. *Journal of Consulting and Clinical Psychology, 75*(3), 475–488. https://doi.org/10.1037/0022-006X.75.3.475

Walsh, B. T., Seidman, S. N., Sysko, R., & Gould, M. (2002). Placebo response in studies of major depression: Variable, substantial, and growing. *JAMA, 287*(14), 1840–1847. https://doi.org/10.1001/jama.287.14.1840

Wartberg, L., Kriston, L., & Thomasius, R. (2018). Depressive symptoms in adolescents – Prevalence and associated psychosocial features in a representative sample. *Deutsches Ärzteblatt, 115*, 549–555. https://doi.org/10.3238/arztebl.2018.0549

Wise, L. A., Zierler, S., Krieger, N., & Harlow, B. L. (2001). Adult onset of major depressive disorder in relation to early life violent victimisation: A case-control study. *Lancet, 358*(9285), 881–887. https://doi.org/10.1016/S0140-6736(01)06072-X

Witt, A., Brown, R., Plener, P. L., Brähler, E., Fegert, J. M., & Clemens, V. (2019a). Kindes-misshandlung und deren Langzeitfolgen – Analyse einer repräsentativen deutschen Stichprobe. *Zeitschrift für Psychiatrie, Psychologie und Psychotherapie, 67*(2), 100–111. https://doi.org/10.1024/1661-4747/a000378

Witt, A., Sachser, C., Plener, P. L., Brähler, E., & Fegert, J. M. (2019b). The prevalence and consequences of adverse childhood experiences in the German population. *Deutsches Ärzteblatt, 116*, 635–642. https://doi.org/10.3238/arztebl.2019.0635

World Health Organization. (1992). *The ICD-10 classification of mental and behavioural disorders: Clinical descriptions and diagnostic guidelines*. World Health Organization. https://apps.who.int/iris/handle/10665/37958

World Health Organization. (2004). *The global burden disease: 2004 update*. https://www.who.int/healthinfo/global_burden_disease/GBD_report_2004update_full.pdf

World Health Organization. (2017). *Depression and other common mental health disorders*. Global Health Estimates. https://who.int/mental_health/management/depression/prevalence_global_health_estimates/en

Wöller, W. (2006). *Trauma und Persönlichkeitsstörungen: Psychodynamisch-integrative Therapie (PITT)*. Schattauer.

Wolpe, J. (1969). *The practice of behavior therapy* (2nd ed.). Pergamon Press.

Memory Work—A New Method for the Treatment of Depression: EMDR Therapy

1

EMDR Therapy as a New Treatment Approach

Maria Lehnung and Michael Hase

Things are only past when they don't hurt anymore.
—Anonymous

INTRODUCTION

The cornerstone of our new concept of treating depressive disorders is eye movement desensitization and reprocessing (EMDR) therapy. EMDR therapy is a psychotherapy approach that was developed by Francine Shapiro, PhD, in 1987 and it has proven its efficacy in treating posttraumatic stress disorder (PTSD). EMDR is recognized worldwide as one of the most effective treatments for PTSD. Unlike the usual forms of talking therapy, EMDR is based on a completely different neurobiological mechanism that was discovered and documented by a Korean research group (Baek et al., 2019). To understand the processes that occurred during EMDR treatment and to improve treatment planning, the Adaptive Information Processing (AIP) Model was hypothesized and the concept of biologically active, pathogenic memories, that can be traumatic and non-traumatic, were developed. In this chapter, EMDR therapy and its basic concepts, as well as the first pioneering publication in the field of depression, are discussed.

HISTORY OF EMDR THERAPY

Francine Shapiro developed EMDR therapy, a new method of psychotherapy, in 1987.
Shapiro, an American psychologist and researcher, made the discovery that when she focused on a very distressing experience that was bothering her, she found that her eyes moved back and forth, rapidly in saccadic movements and, to her surprise, her distress decreased! Being a great observer of human behavior, she thought it interesting and repeatedly tried it again on herself, with similar results. She thought this discovery was so meaningful that she

tried it out with other people and then conducted the first scientific study on eye movement and desensitization (EMD) as it was called then. The population for this analysis included traumatized Vietnam veterans and victims of rape. After the EMD intervention, the clients reported a considerable reduction in the intensity of trauma-associated memories and of their subjective experience of stress caused by these memories. In 1989, the *Journal of Traumatic Stress Studies* published Shapiro's paper "Efficacy of the Eye Movement Desensitization Procedure in the Treatment of Traumatic Memories." The article elicited a response in the psychotherapeutic world, and Shapiro developed her approach further. It was the beginning of the development of EMDR therapy. From the outset, Shapiro emphasized the importance of scientific backing and research of this method, including its efficacy and the factors responsible for this effect.

WHAT IS EMDR ACTUALLY?

EMDR is a treatment for processing stressful memories that cause psychological and psychosomatic disorders. EMDR therapy is based on the AIP system—a particular model of pathogenesis and change. The AIP system says that people are capable of adaptively processing incidents, even ones that are severe and distressing. However, for various reasons it is possible that this natural process can get stuck. The event then becomes dysfunctional and is stored in fragments. This EMDR approach helps jumpstart the AIP system so that the person can reprocess the distressing experience in spite of this disruption. It is essentially a person's system for self-healing, which leads to the resolution of the symptoms from which the patient was previously suffering. The central elements of the reprocessing include focusing on the distressing event, as well as alternating bilateral stimulation.

THE ADAPTIVE INFORMATION PROCESSING MODEL OF EMDR THERAPY

EMDR therapy is based on the AIP Model. AIP assumes that a past stressful or traumatic experience is not integrated as a normal, explicit memory; instead, it is stored as an implicit, dysfunctional, trauma-memory network. Indeed, neurobiological research shows that many findings support this assumption (Yehuda et al., 2015). Studies show that when an unprocessed traumatic memory was recalled, cortical structures of long-term memory were not activated, as would be expected. Instead, for the most part, limbic structures were activated. In their 2007 case study, Jatzko and Ruf observed that when placing a patient who had been in a severe motor vehicle accident in an fMRI, while simultaneously confronting the patient with a few short sentences from a recording of the accident, areas in the cingulate gyrus and in the tertiary visual cortex were activated. Frontal areas were deactivated during this time. Van der Kolk et al. (2003) and Pagani et al. (2012) made the same observation that traumatic memories were not stored where old memories would normally be found in the brain.

EMDR has the goal of processing these stuck, implicit, dysfunctional trauma networks so that the memories can be integrated and the pathology can be resolved. Indeed, this has also been demonstrated in neurobiology. In the case study by Jatzko and Ruf (2007), the patient was treated with EMDR. After the treatment, the patient again underwent an fMRI scan. The biological traces that had previously been observed in the limbic system, as well as in the tertiary visual cortex, had now disappeared and were no longer dysfunctional; they were integrated. Pagani et al. (2012) found a similar result in his EEG study.

The AIP Model is fundamentally a resource-oriented model. It starts from the premise that a person is capable of processing experiences through the use of an internal system of information processing that is very likely located in the central nervous system. In a processing system of this kind, important things are remembered and unimportant things are deleted (forgotten). Information that has been previously stored in cortical long-term memory is changed by more current information in this process of *information processing*. This is similar to the situation where a stressful life experience changes over time and becomes less painful as new knowledge and life experiences are gained. It can be assumed that some of this natural information processing occurs during the course of the day, but that significant portions take place during the REM and non-REM phases of sleep (Stickgold et al., 2001). Under certain conditions, the information processing system is disrupted or blocked in its functioning. These memories then remain stored in a raw, unprocessed, state-specific form. These dysfunctionally stored memories are the cause of mental and psychosomatic disorders and are also called *pathogenic memories* (Centonze et al., 2005).

These memories are frequently organized in memory networks—around elements such as a primary affect, people involved, and so forth. Shapiro's assumption (2018) is that if this kind of unprocessed memory is not spontaneously processed in the time period shortly after the experience, it is stored as if frozen and isolated from adaptive information. After this initial time following the stressful or traumatic event, it either does not change or only changes to a small degree without therapeutic intervention (Shapiro, 2018).

If a dysfunctionally stored, unprocessed memory of this kind is activated, it has a strong influence on reality and somehow feels *real*, as if it is happening right now. Often, patients experience intrusions—typical symptoms of PTSD. Nonetheless, other dysfunctionally stored memories can be expressed as pain symptoms, an intrusive emotion in the case of affective disorders, or a cognitive intrusion such as a dysfunctional belief. When the information processing system is activated, through focusing and then bilateral stimulation, the memory is reprocessed, primarily with eye movements. Clinically, the result is the end of symptoms and normalization of behavior(s).

PATHOGENIC MEMORIES

Primarily, EMDR has been proven effective in the treatment of PTSD (Khan et al., 2018; Schulz et al., 2015; World Health Organization [WHO], 2013). However, there are several publications that demonstrate the efficacy of EMDR in the processing of other forms of memory. Out of the vast literature on this subject, preliminarily, we will focus on the studies of Cvetek (2008) and Frustaci et al. (2010). Both studies show that processing adverse life experiences that do not meet the Criterion A standard for PTSD (mortal danger) can lead also to a clinical improvement in patients that is measurable via appropriate tools. For example, Frustaci et al. (2010) showed via the measurement of heart rate variability that the changes that occur through EMDR reprocessing encompass not only mental changes but adjustments in the autonomic nervous system. This corresponds to clinical experience that shows that pain disorders and psychosomatic symptoms can be successfully treated with EMDR therapy. Therefore, we can assume that PTSD is only a special case of a *memory processing disorder*.

In a research article on the neurobiology of psychotherapy, Centonze and his collaborators indicated that implicit traumatic memories and non-traumatic memories are of great concern for both healthy and dysfunctional brain functioning (Centonze et al., 2005). According to Centonze, these memories store the sensory fragments of the experience and they are not only *remembered*, but are biologically active. We can see their biological activity in intrusions, such as in PTSD. These pathogenic memories are similar to Shapiro's dysfunctionally stored memories and can clinically be seen in the following cases:

- Traumatic memory may lead to the symptoms of PTSD.
- Addiction memory may lead to cravings.
- Pain memory in somebody who lost a limb may suffer from phantom pain.
- Stressful attachment memory or depression memory may lead to the symptoms of depression, such as cognitive intrusions in terms of dysfunctional beliefs.

In other words, Centonze and his collaborators, who are not involved in EMDR therapy, describe the AIP Model of EMDR therapy! Hase et al. (2017) concluded that it made sense to introduce the following ideas into psychotherapy concerning pathogenic memories: they are the cause of mental and psychosomatic disorders; they can be understood within the framework of the AIP Model of EMDR therapy; and they can be treated with the protocols and procedures of EMDR. EMDR therapy's AIP Model and the Pathogenic Memories Model come from different branches of psychotherapy. In this way, knowledge gained from clinical practice and theoretical research converge and complement each other.

It still remains for us to answer the question of how a blockage or impairment of a person's intrinsic ability to process these memories comes about. Here, there are several possibilities to consider. In PTSD, we see a massive, intense experience, that can also be assumed in the case of some pain disorders. This *impact* leads to the formation of an implicit memory. As Hofmann convincingly portrays in another section of this book, a humiliating event, verbal violence, or rejection from one's peer group also can have a serious effect at vulnerable times of mental development. Therefore, the formation of a pathogenic memory does not always require experiences that fulfill the classic criteria of a posttraumatic stress in terms of the diagnostic manuals, such as the *International Classification of Diseases* or the *Diagnostic and Statistical Manual of Mental Disorders*.

Another way to create a pathogenic memory could be frequently experiencing certain maladaptive/negative conditions. Regardless of how a depression develops, the repeated experience of depression could itself lead to the formation of an implicit dysfunctionally stored memory (e.g., a memory of the condition of the body during depression) that can then be triggered, activated, and expressed once again in a depressive experience, without any of this actually corresponding to a current depressive episode. In this context, we use the term *states* as a meaning derived from the AIP Model. States—from an AIP perspective—are memory fragments and do not mean the same thing as the ego states described by Federn (1952; Horowitz, 1979).

It can be assumed that both paths of development are not exclusive, but can occur in combination. Note that information processing impairments are not only found in the occurrence itself but in individual factors, such as the absence of internal preparation for an occurrence, age or *immaturity* issues, insufficient knowledge, or physical weakness.

Until now, an important aspect has gone unmentioned. Since the appearance of the first edition of Shapiro's 1995 textbook, she emphasized that adaptive information must be available and able to be activated in order to reprocess the memory. In the various editions of her textbooks and training manuals, she formulated and fleshed out these thoughts in different ways. It became clear that Shapiro understood the AIP Model not only as the model of unprocessed memory, but also as the model of adaptive information, of positive memories. These are normally called *resources* in EMDR therapy. Reprocessing begins when patients have adequate resources with the ability to access them so that they can stay within their window of tolerance. There are numerous resources that therapists use. However, Shapiro emphasized that focus should be on using the least amount of resources to ensure staying in the patient's window of tolerance and to make sure that state change interventions such as resources were not being used instead of reprocessing. According to Amano and Toichi (2016), slowly stimulating a resource makes it easier to access positive emotion that shows a different activity pattern than the faster-paced processing of dysfunctional material. Further research into the targeted use of resources appears promising in the context of many disorders. The use of the AIP Model supports accessing the *nodes* (pathogenic memories) driving the symptoms of depressive patients, resulting in a clear and practical plan for treatment. At the same time, the patient's resources are accessed. The patient's symptoms provide important clues about the activity of various networks of unprocessed memory, so that priorities can be set in the treatment plan. The AIP Model directs thought and action in EMDR therapy. This is portrayed in more detail in the chapters on the treatment of depressive patients with the DeprEnd Protocol.

THE EIGHT PHASES OF EMDR THERAPY

EMDR is a therapy in eight treatment segments (8 phases).

First, there is *Phase 1/History Taking*. The main goal is to understand the patient's symptoms using the AIP Model. Deal with the past by asking: *What happened? Which events triggered the disorder? What are the dysfunctionally processed memories?* Address the present with the question: *Which events, situations, and circumstances trigger the symptoms today?* Formulate concerns for the future by inquiring: *How are the patient's perspectives on their future distorted by these memories?*

In *Phase 2*, we focus on stabilizing the patient, to the extent it is necessary, and preparing them for EMDR treatment. The stabilization is done individually, depending on the patient's situation. Resources can include physical stabilization, psychosocial stabilization, or mental stabilization. Usually, mental stabilization has priority, since EMDR is overwhelmingly used in the context of psychotherapy.

How much stabilization a patient needs and which methods should be used are dependent on the patient's needs. The following tenet is used to inform treatment: Use only the resources needed to support moving into the reprocessing phases. In order to evaluate this need, use these four tests to assess patient readiness.

- *Everyday Life Test:* With the Everyday Life Test, we look at the level of functioning patients have in everyday life. Can they still maintain the most important functions of everyday life when under stress? How much affect tolerance do patients have? How do they respond when under stress with their partner, their child, their place of work?
- *Safe Place Test:* The Safe Place Test is used to assess whether patients can experience and tolerate a positive resource for a short period of time.

- *Stimulation Test:* The Stimulation Test is used to evaluate how patients respond to a series of bilateral eye movements. Can they tolerate it well?
- *History-Taking Test:* The History-Taking Test reveals if patients can report the narrative of their distressing experiences without decompensating.

If all four tests have a positive result, proceed to Phase 3. If patients have difficulty with some tests, more stabilization is needed.

Other functions of Phase 2 are to explain EMDR therapy, and coordinate a treatment plan with patients that include the order of how dysfunctional memories will be processed.

In *Phase 3* of EMDR therapy, we work with a specific, dysfunctionally stored memory that we have identified earlier. This phase is called the *Assessment Phase*. Here, a memory is activated by asking for its components such as the image, positive cognition (PC) and negative cognition (NC), affects, and sensations. At first, patients are asked to focus on a specific image that captures the worst part of the memory. Next, the NCs and PCs are elicited that also connect with the memory. The negative belief is a cognitive schema that is a negative statement about the self that is irrational, charged with affect, and often generalizable. The goal of activating the NC is to access the negative affect and elicit the positive memory networks in the form of the PC by saying: *What would you prefer to believe about yourself instead of* (state the NC)? It is then rated on a scale of 1 to 7: *When you think of that memory, how true do the words* (repeat the PC) *feel to you now on a scale of 1 to 7, where 1 feels completely false and 7 feels completely true?* This number is the *Validity of Cognition (VOC)*, which in the course of the treatment with EMDR normally increases toward 7 without direct cognitive work.

The NC opens the gate to access the affect associated with the memory. We ask about this affect, so that we can monitor the changes that occur during EMDR treatment. This is recorded and measured by Joseph Wolpe's scale *Subjective Units of Disturbance* (SUD; Wolpe, 1958). Finally, the distress/sensation is located in the body. At this point, the dysfunctionally stored memory is fully activated and we can proceed to the bilateral stimulation and reprocessing that is Phase 4.

Phase 4/Desensitization Phase is where desensitization and reprocessing occur. During this phase, bilateral stimulation is used, usually in the form of eye movements. EMDR therapy processing allows for the unique way each patient has stored information. In this process, many changes can occur, for example, in each of the modalities, patients may have different experiences. Images may come in the foreground and become fainter or more detailed, or appear and disappear; affects are elicited and can change; and physical sensations may come into consciousness as the body remembers. Over time, this process moves toward an adaptive integration of the memory.

When the original event no longer feels distressing, the PC—that by now is seen as more true—is strengthened and installed again using eye movements. This installation is called *Phase 5/Installation Phase*.

In *Phase 6/Body Scan Phase*, patients pay attention to what is happening in their bodies to check for any unresolved issues. Patients bring whatever is left of the memory paired with the previously installed PC to mind, which has already been installed, as they scan their entire body. If no unpleasant physical sensation is noticed, the process is completed. If an unpleasant physical sensation occurs, it is then reprocessed with eye movements until it decreases or goes away.

Phase 7 is the *Closure Phase* of the therapy session. Patients are told that the reprocessing may continue after the session. They are instructed to notice new insights, thoughts, memories, physical sensations, or dreams and to jot down what they notice to go over at the next session.

The *Reevaluation Phase* or *Phase 8* occurs in the next session. Progress is checked to figure out what is next in the treatment plan. The patient and therapist discuss the subsequent treatment together.

THE MECHANISM OF ACTION OF EMDR

For a long time, the mechanism of action of EMDR therapy remained uncertain but over the past few years, it has been investigated from various perspectives. As is the case for other psychotherapies, it is probable that there is not just one mechanism of action for EMDR, but rather different mechanisms in its various phases. Landin-Romero and his collaborators (2018) summarize these studies on the mechanisms of action for EMDR. They review and differentiate the psychological models from the psychophysiological models as well as the neurobiological models.

Early in the history of EMDR, Dyck (1993) presented the orienting response hypothesis. According to this hypothesis, EMDR triggers an orienting reaction—when there is a new stimulus, a reaction occurs resulting in an elevated arousal and de-synchronization of electric activity in the brain. Habituation occurs after multiple exposures to the stimulus in the absence of a dangerous situation. Then, the orienting response gives way to a relaxation response. As habituation continues, it leads to a synchronization of slow brain waves in the limbic system and this is associated with a safe feeling.

Baddeley and Hitch (1974) present a different psychological model called the Working Memory Hypothesis. It postulates that there is a central executive system responsible for the integration of information that is stored in various subordinate systems; for example, the visuo-spatial sketchpad and the phonological loop. If a second task, such as eye movements, is conducted during the recall of information, there are fewer resources available for recalling the content of the memory and its quality decreases. According to the theory, through this process, the memory fades and is less distressing, and the traumatic experience loses its traumatic qualities. A number of studies point in this direction.

At the beginning of EMDR research, psychophysiological models also played a big role. Francine Shapiro's assumption was that the eye movements and dual attention that occur during EMDR lead to specific psychophysiological changes that form the foundation for the treatment's efficacy. Studies (Sack et al, 2008; Wilson et al., 1996) showed that eye movements lead to measurable physiological changes such as decreases in skin conductance, heart rate, and stimulation of the parasympathetic nervous system, which explains a de-arousal during and after EMDR treatment. Later, neurobiological models demonstrated that structural and functional changes in the brain are associated with EMDR (Bossini et al., 2011).

In their complex EEG study during Phase 3/Assessment, Pagani and his collaborators (2012) showed that limbic structures as well as tertiary visual cortex structures were active. During bilateral stimulation, structures were activated in the frontal brain lobe—especially in the orbitofrontal cortex—and interacted with limbic structures. Pagani and his collaborators interpreted this interaction of the two systems as a sign of processing occurring. When they tested patients an hour later, they found that the active structures then were mostly large associative networks in the left temporo-occipital region. They concluded that this was a sign that the previously unprocessed memory was now successfully processed.

In 2019, Baek and his colleagues used an animal model to provide evidence for the primary mechanism of action for EMDR at a cellular level. Due to its scientific importance and good research methodology, the journal *Nature* published the article. Using classic conditioning, Baek et al. taught mice to fear a sound. As expected, the classically conditioned fear induced by electric shocks disappeared with repeated exposure to the sound when not accompanied by electric shocks. Rather than just working with this one paradigm (mice get used to the repeated sound), they also exposed a group of mice not only to the sound, but also to bilateral stimulation that was supplied with LEDs alternating between left and right. The light strip was always running at the point the mice were looking at—a form of mouse EMDR. This EMDR was shown to be most effective at reducing the fear reaction (conditioned stimulus [CS] + EMDR; see Figure 1.1). It was markedly more effective than exposure alone (CS).

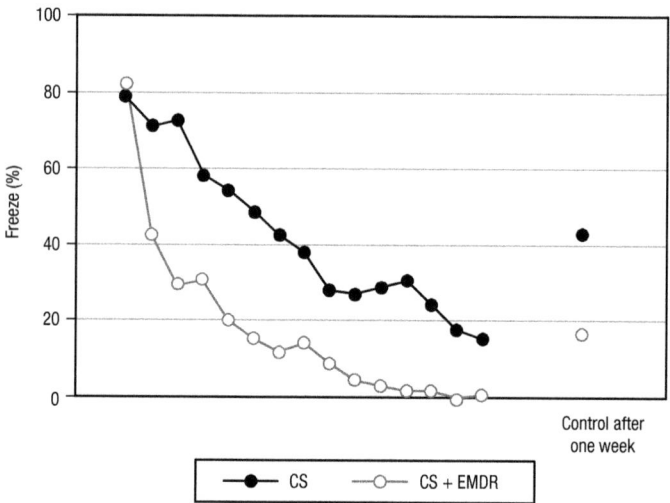

FIGURE 1.1. Efficacy of exposure versus EMDR in the mouse experiment. Reduction of fear (freezing) with exposure to the sound (CS) and exposure to the sound with added eye movements (CS + EMDR).

CS, conditioned stimulus; EMDR, eye movement desensitization and reprocessing.

Source: Data from Baek, J., Lee, S., Cho, T., Kim, S. W., Kim, M., Yoon, Y., Kim, K. K., Byun, J., Kim, S. J., Jeong, J., & Shin, H. S. (2019). Neural circuits underlying a psychotherapeutic regimen for fear disorders. *Nature, 566*(7744), 339–343. https://doi.org/10.1038/s41586-019-0931-y

The results were that the combination of exposure to the sound and alternating bilateral stimulation led to the clearest and most sustained reduction of the fear reaction.

Baek et al. (2019) additionally investigated the path in the brain that leads to this accelerated reduction of fear during eye movements by using neuronal single-cell recordings. In this recording, single cells are punctured and the electrical activity is measured along the path of assumed neuronal activity. They found that the combination of exposure and bilateral stimulation first activates the superior colliculus (Figure 1.2). After this, the mediodorsal thalamus

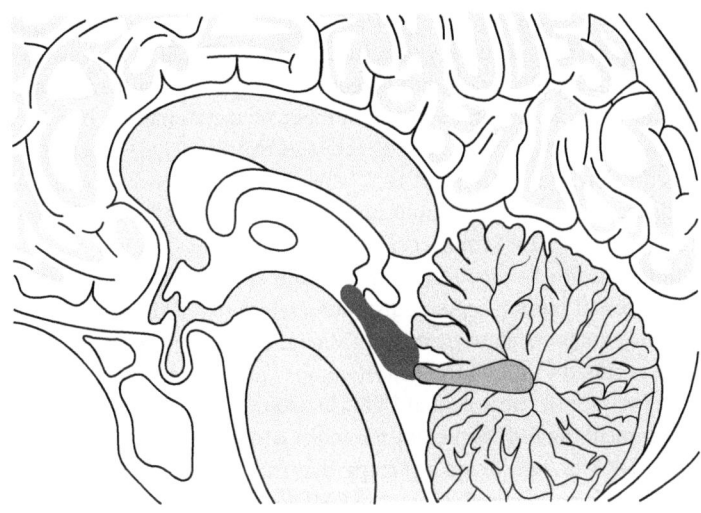

FIGURE 1.2. The anatomical position of the corpora quadrigemina and the colliculi superiori (in black) in the human brain.

is activated. The activity of these two centers makes it possible to predict to what degree the fear reaction would decrease. If the thalamus was prevented from firing, there was no reduction of the fear reaction. If the neurons of the superior colliculus did not fire, there was also no reduction of the fear reaction. The communication between these two regions is necessary for the reduction of the fear response.

How does this communication lead to a decline in the fear reaction? Baek et al. found that the combined procedures of exposure and alternating bilateral stimulation (mouse EMDR) reduced the reaction of activating neurons (sometimes called fear neurons) in the basolateral amygdala. Here, there is a two-step inhibition process between the mediodorsal thalamus and the basolateral amygdala. This process was more effective than all other forms of stimulation, including exposure by itself.

These studies have great importance for explaining the mechanism of action of EMDR as they explain sufficiently and comprehensively the effects of EMDR, at least as used on mice. Exposure and alternating bilateral stimulation activate a neuronal path that connects the superior colliculus and the mediodorsal thalamus, that then inhibits the fear reaction in the basolateral amygdala. Exposure to the fear stimulus alone or alternating bilateral stimulation alone do not inhibit the fear response to the same extent as the combination of both does. In the study, it was also shown that simultaneous and other stimulations are less effective than alternating bilateral stimulation. In summary, the work of Baek et al. seems to have identified one of the main neurobiological mechanisms of EMDR therapy.

From the beginning, EMDR therapy was shown to be a very successful form of therapy, especially for treating PTSD, and encouraged research. Up until the end of the 1980s, PTSD was considered difficult or impossible to treat. It is why it was so surprising that after four to six sessions of EMDR, many studies showed that patients with simple PTSD were free of PTSD at a rate of 80%; the results remained stable over 3 years. For complex

PTSD, EMDR is more effective than medication (Van der Kolk et al., 2007). For children and adolescents, EMDR is also very effective. In total, EMDR is at least as effective as trauma-focused behavioral therapy, but it requires 40% fewer hours of treatment (Power et al., 2002; Van Etten & Taylor, 1998). A number of meta-analyses have demonstrated that trauma-focused therapies are most effective at treating PTSD especially EMDR and trauma-focused behavioral therapy. In fact, where there is comorbidity in patients, these conditions significantly improve without needing to be a direct focus of treatment (Chen et al., 2015; Khan et al., 2018; Schulz et al., 2015).

The National Health Service (NHS) in England showed in their investigation of the cost-effectiveness of all trauma-centered psychotherapies that EMDR therapy was an effective and cost-efficient approach to treatment (Mavranezouli et al., 2020). For this reason, in 2013, EMDR was added to the *WHO Guidelines for the Management of Conditions Specifically Related to Stress* for the treatment of PTSD in adults. There are many other international guidelines recommending EMDR therapy for adults and children.

At first, EMDR was considered a therapy that was first and foremost effective for the treatment of PTSD. If one takes a closer look at EMDR therapy, however, it becomes clear that the AIP Model can be applied to other disorders. This is because these disorders are caused by, partially caused by, or made worse by dysfunctionally processed memories. Currently, many studies confirm the efficacy of EMDR for many other disorders.

The disease model based on the AIP Model works for pain disorders as well. Frequently experiencing a biological pain condition, such as migraines or phantom pain, leads to the formation of a pain memory. After processing of the triggering distressing memories, pain memories, and trauma-related pain memories with EMDR, the pain is reduced considerably or disappears completely (Ghanbari et al., 2018; Maroufi et al., 2016; Rostaminejad et al., 2017; Tesarz et al., 2014). Even for anxiety disorders, often triggered by distressing experiences (e.g., dental fear, fear of dogs, test anxiety), many investigations show that EMDR therapy is effective (Cook-Vienot & Taylor, 2012; Doering et al., 2013). Furthermore, there is a controlled study on the efficacy of EMDR for the treatment of relapses for alcoholic patients, in which patients focused on drug-specific memories (Hase et al., 2008; Kuijer et al., 2020). For all these issues and disorders that extend beyond classic PTSD, there is nonetheless the need for further systematic studies in order to strengthen the findings already made in the existing studies.

EMDR IN THE TREATMENT OF DEPRESSIVE DISORDERS

Depression is one of the most frequent mental disorders that we encounter and EMDR therapy was used early on for the treatment of depression. Francine Shapiro published a case in which she treated a depressive mother with EMDR. Mia, the patient, had lost her 12-year-old child in an accident. She became depressive as a consequence and attempted suicide. Shapiro treated her with three sessions of EMDR, and afterward the depression remitted (Shapiro & Silk Forrest, 1997). Additionally, in Philip Manfield's book *Extending EMDR*, he writes about two cases of depressive patients who were treated successfully with EMDR (Manfield, 1998). Altogether there is a large body of literature and case studies of depressive patients treated with EMDR that has been compiled and analyzed elsewhere excellently (Luber, 2016).

Chapter 1 EMDR Therapy as a New Treatment Approach

In 2008, Bae, Kim, and Park published a small case series on the treatment of depression with EMDR. They treated two adolescent patients; one of the patients was 16 years old. Her father had died 1 year earlier and, afterward, she decompensated at her boarding school. She was treated with EMDR in three sessions. The focus of these sessions was the death of her father and the future. Her depression scores fell considerably, and at the end of 4 weeks of therapy, as well as in the follow-up after 12 weeks, she had no more depressive symptoms.

The second patient in this case series was a 14-year-old girl whose father had separated from the family and she had to leave her school. She developed a major depression, lost a considerable amount of weight, and had suicidal ideation. She was treated with six sessions of EMDR. The focus was on the friends she had lost, her father's affair, and her fears about the future. Here, the depression also completely remitted and the result was still stable at her follow-up after 3 months.

The study by Bae, Kim, and Park (2008), along with our own successful retrospective study on EMDR therapy and depression, provided us with significant encouragement to conduct further studies of our own on the use of EMDR therapy for depressive disorders. Our additional studies that followed then led to the European Depression EMDR Network (EDEN) study conducted by our European research group. These studies are described in the next chapters.

REFERENCES

Amano, T., & Toichi, M. (2016). The role of alternating bilateral stimulation in establishing positive cognition in EMDR therapy: A multi-channel near-infrared spectroscopy study. *PLoS ONE, 11*(10), e0162735. https://doi.org/10.1371/journal.pone.0162735

Baddeley, A. D., & Hitch, G. J. L. (1974). Working memory. In G. A. Bower (Ed.), *The psychology of learning and motivation: Advances in research and theory* (pp. 47–89). Academic Press.

Bae, H., Kim, D., & Park, Y. C. (2008) Eye movement desensitization and reprocessing for adolescent depression. *Psychiatry Investigation 5*(1), 60–65. https://doi.org/10.4306/pi.2008.5.1.60

Baek, J., Lee, S. W., Cho, T., Kim, S. W., Kim, M., Yoon, Y., Kim, K. K., Byun, J., Kim, S. J., Jeong, J., & Shin, H. S. (2019). Neural circuits underlying a psychotherapeutic regimen for fear disorders. *Nature, 566*(7744), 339–343. https://doi.org/10.1038/s41586-019-0931-y

Bossini, L., Tavanti, M., Calossi, S., Polizzotto, N. R., Vatti, G., Marino, D., & Castrogiovanni, P. (2011). EMDR treatment for posttraumatic stress disorder, with focus on hippocampal volumes: A pilot study. *Journal of Neuropsychiatry and Clinical Neurosciences, 23*(2), E1–E2. https://doi.org/10.1176/jnp.23.2.jnpe1

Centonze, D., Siracusano, A., Calabresi, P., & Bernardi, G. (2005). Removing pathogenic memories: A neurobiology of psychotherapy. *Molecular Psychiatry, 32*(2), 123–132. https://doi.org/10.1385/MN:32:2:123

Chen, L., Zhang, G., Hu, M., & Liang, X. (2015). Eye movement desensitization and reprocessing versus cognitive-behavioral therapy for adult posttraumatic stress disorder: Systematic review and meta-analysis. *Journal of Nervous and Mental Disease, 203*(6), 443–451. https://doi.org/10.1097/NMD.0000000000000306

Cook-Vienot, R., & Taylor, R. J. (2012). Comparison of eye movement desensitization and reprocessing and biofeedback/stress inoculation training in treating test anxiety. *Journal of EMDR Practice and Research, 6*(2), 62–72. https://doi.org/10.1891/1933-3196.6.2.62

Cvetek, R. (2008). EMDR treatment of distressful experiences that fail to meet the criteria for PTSD. *Journal of EMDR Practice and Research, 2*(1), 2–14. https://doi.org/10.1891/1933-3196.2.1.2

Doering, S., Ohlmeier, M. C., de Jongh, A., Hofmann, A., & Bisping, V. (2013). Efficacy of a trauma-focused treatment approach for dental phobia: A randomized clinical trial. *European Journal of Oral Sciences, 121*(6), 584–593. https://doi.org/10.1111/eos.12090

Dyck, M. J. (1993). A proposal for a conditioning model of eye movement desensitization treatment for posttraumatic stress disorder. *Journal of Behavior Therapy and Experimental Psychiatry, 24*, 201–210. https://doi.org/10.1016/0005-7916(93)90022-o

Federn, P. (1952). *Ego psychology and the psychoses*. Basic Books.

Frustaci, A., Lanza. G., Fernandez, I., di Giannantonio, M., & Pozzi, G. (2010). Changes in psychological symptoms and heart rate variability during EMDR treatment: A case series of subthreshold PTSD. *Journal of EMDR Research and Practice, 2*, 26–40. https://doi.org/10.1891/1933-3196.4.1.3

Ghanbari, N., Afrasiabifar, A., & Behnammoghadam, M. (2018). Comparing the effect of eye movement desensitization and reprocessing (EMDR) with guided imagery on pain severity in patients with rheumatoid arthritis. *Journal of Pain Research, 11*, 2107–2113. https://doi.org/10.2147/JPR.S158981

Hase, M., Schallmayer, S., & Sack, M. (2008). EMDR reprocessing of the addiction memory: Pretreatment, posttreatment, and 1-month follow-up. *Journal of EMDR Practice and Research, 2*, 170–179. https://doi.org/10.1891/1933-3196.2.3.170

Hase, M., Balmaceda, U. M., Ostacoli, L., Liebermann, P., & Hofmann, A. (2017). The AIP model of EMDR therapy and pathogenic memories. *Frontiers in Psychology, 8*, 1578. https://doi.org/10.3389/fpsyg.2017.01578

Horowitz, M. (1979). *States of mind: Analysis of change in psychotherapy*. Plenum Medical Book Company.

Jatzko, A., & Ruf, M. (2007). *Durch EMDR normalisierte funktionelle Verarbeitungspro-zesse bei PTBS – eine fMRT Pilotstudie*. Poster presented at the DeGPT Conference 2007, Basel, Switzerland.

Khan, A. M., Dar, S., Ahmed, R., Bachu, R., Adnan, M., & Kotapati, V. P. (2018, September). Cognitive behavioral therapy versus eye movement desensitization and reprocessing in patients with posttraumatic stress disorder: systematic review and meta-analysis of randomized clinical trials. *Cureus 10*(9), e3250. https://doi.org/10.7759/cureus.3250

Kuijer, E. J., Ferragud, A., & Milton, A. L. (2020). Retrieval extinction and relapse prevention: Rewriting maladaptive drug memories? *Frontiers in Behavioral Neuroscience, 14*, 23. https://doi.org/10.3389/fnbeh.2020.00023

Landin-Romero, R., Moreno-Alcazar, A., Pagani, M., & Amann, B. L. (2018). How does eye movement desensitization and reprocessing therapy work? A systematic review on suggested mechanisms of action. *Frontiers in Psychology, 9*, 1395. https://doi.org/10.3389/fpsyg.2018.01395

Luber, M. (2016). EMDR therapy and mood disorders. In M. Luber (Ed.), *EMDR therapy scripted protocols and summary sheets: Treating anxiety, obsessive-compulsive, mood-related conditions* (pp. 213–222). Springer Publishing Company.

Manfield, P. (Ed.). (1998). *Extending EMDR: A casebook of innovative applications*. W. W. Norton & Company.

Maroufi, M., Zamani, S., Izadikah, Z., Marofi, M., & O'Connor, P. (2016). Investigating the effect of eye movement desensitization and reprocessing (EMDR) on postoperative pain intensity in adolescents undergoing surgery: A randomized controlled trial. *Journal of Advanced Nursing, 72*(9), 2207–2217. https://doi.org/10.1111/jan.12985

Mavranezouli, I., Megnin-Viggars, O., Daly, C., Dias, S., Welton, N. J., Stockton, S., Bhutani, G., Grey, N., Leach, J., Greenberg, N., Katona, C., El-Leithy, S., & Pilling, S. (2020). Psychological treatments for post-traumatic stress disorder in adults: A network meta-analysis. *Psychological Medicine, 50*(4), 542–555. https://doi.org/10.1017/S0033291720000070

Pagani, M., Di Lorenzo, G., Verardo, A. R., Nicolais, G., Monaco, L., Lauretti, G., Russo, R., Niolu, C., Ammaniti, M., Fernandez, I., & Siracusano, A. (2012). Neurobiological correlates of EMDR monitoring – An EEG study. *PLoS ONE, 7*(9), e45753. https://doi.org/10.1371/journal.pone.0045753

Power, K., McGoldrick, T., Brown, K., Buchanan, R., Sharp, D., Swanson, V., & Karatzias, A. (2002). A controlled comparison of eye movement desensitization and reprocessing versus exposure plus cognitive restructuring versus waiting list in the treatment of post-traumatic stress disorder. *Clinical Psychology and Psychotherapy, 9*(5), 299–318. https://doi.org/10.1002/cpp.341

Rostaminejad, A., Behnammoghadam, M., Rostaminejad, M., Behnammoghadam, Z., & Bashti, S. (2017). Efficacy of eye movement desensitization and reprocessing on the phantom limb pain of patients with amputations within a 24-month follow-up. *International Journal of Rehabilitation Research, 40*(3), 209–214. https://doi.org/10.1097/MRR.0000000000000227

Sack, M., Lempa, W., Steinmetz, A., Lamprecht, F., & Hofmann, A. (2008). Alterations in autonomic tone during trauma exposure using eye movement desensitization and reprocessing (EMDR) – Results of a preliminary investigation. *Journal of Anxiety Disorders, 22*(7), 1264–1271. https://doi.org/10.1016/j.janxdis.2008.01.007

Schulz, S., Dahm, A., Herrmann-Frank, A., Martinsohn-Schittkowski, W., Nocon, M., & Sühlfleisch-Thurau, U. (2015). EMDR – Eine Methode wird anerkannt. *Deutsches Aerzteblatt, 13*(01), 34–36. https://www.aerzteblatt.de/archiv/167152

Shapiro, F. (1989). Efficacy of the eye movement desensitization procedure in the treatment of traumatic memories. *Journal of Traumatic Stress Studies, 2*, 199–223. https://doi.org/10.1002/jts.2490020207

Shapiro, F. (1995). *Eye movement desensitization and reprocessing: Basic principles, protocols and procedures* (1st ed.). Guilford Press.

Shapiro, F. (2018). *Eye movement desensitization and reprocessing (EMDR) therapy: Basic principles, protocols and procedure* (3rd ed.). Guilford Press.

Shapiro, F., & Silk Forrest, M. (1997). *EMDR: The breakthrough therapy for overcoming anxiety, stress, and trauma*. Basic Books.

Stickgold, R., Hobson, J. A., Fosse, R., & Fosse, M. (2001). Sleep, learning, and dreams: Off-line memory reprocessing. *Science, 294*(5544), 1052–1057. https://doi.org/10.1126/science.1063530

Tesarz, J., Leisner, S., Gerhardt, A., Janke, S., Seidler, G. H., Eich, W., & Hartmann, M. (2014). Effects of eye movement desensitization and reprocessing (EMDR) treatment in chronic pain patients: A systematic review. *Pain Medicine, 15*(2), 247–263. https://doi.org/10.1111/pme.12303

Van der Kolk, B. A. (2003). The neurobiology of childhood trauma and abuse. *Child and Adolescent Psychiatric Clinics of North America, 12*(2), 293–317. https://doi.org/10.1016/s1056-4993(03)00003-8

Van der Kolk, B. A., Spinazzola, J., Blaustein, M. E., Hopper, J. W., Hopper, E. K., Korn, D. L., & Simpson, W. B. (2007). A randomized clinical trial of eye movement desensitization and reprocessing (EMDR), fluoxetine, and pill placebo in the treatment of posttraumatic stress disorder: Treatment effects and long-term maintenance. *Journal of Clinical Psychiatry, 68*, 37. https://doi.org/10.4088/jcp.v68n0105

Van Etten, M. L., & Taylor, S. (1998). Comparative efficacy of treatments for post-traumatic stress disorder: A meta-analysis. *Clinical Psychology and Psychotherapy, 5*(3), 126–144. http://dx.doi.org/10.1002/(SICI)1099-0879(199809)5:3<126::AID-CPP153>3.0.CO;2-H

Wilson, D. L., Silver, S. M., Covi, W. G., & Foster, S. J. (1996). Eye movement desensitization and reprocessing: Effectiveness and autonomic correlates. *Journal of Behavior Therapy and Experimental Psychiatry, 27*(3), 219–229. https://doi.org/10.1016/s0005-7916(96)00026-2

World Health Organization. (2013). *Guidelines for the management of conditions specifically related to stress*. World Health Organization. https://www.who.int/publications/i/item/9789241505406

Wolpe, J. (1958). *Psychotherapy by reciprocal inhibition*. Stanford, CA: Stanford University Press.

Yehuda, R., Hoge, C. W., McFarlane, A. C., Vermetten, E., Lanius, R. A., Nievergelt, C. M., Hobfoll, S. E., Koenen K. C., Neylan, T. C., & Hyman, S. E. (2015). Post-traumatic stress disorder. *Nature Reviews Disease Primers, 1*, 15057. https://doi.org/10.1038/nrdp.2015.57

The EMDR DeprEnd Treatment Manual

2

The EMDR Protocol for the Treatment of Depression (DeprEnd)

Michael Hase

INTRODUCTION

In this chapter, an outline of the eye movement desensitization and reprocessing (EMDR) DeprEnd Protocol, as well as the rationale for its interventions, are given. Also, an important instrument to identify some of the pathogenic memories behind the depressive episodes, the Symptom Event Map, is introduced. In EMDR therapy, treatment plans that adhere to formal guidelines are frequently called protocols. In our book, we use both terms—treatment plans and protocols—synonymously. The EMDR DeprEnd treatment manual is the current treatment plan for depression, and it can largely be seen as evidence based. In addition to the steps for treatment and preparation for reprocessing, the protocol contains a sequence for targeting pathogenic memory networks (Hofmann et al., 2016a, 2016b).

SCIENTIFIC BACKGROUND

After many EMDR therapists reported EMDR therapy's efficacy when treating depressive patients over time, in 2006 Arne Hofmann and Michael Hase spearheaded our team and implemented controlled studies. At the same time, we evaluated and discussed knowledge gained from clinical practice in order to create a treatment plan. In the introduction of this book, we already gave an account of the first controlled study of depressive patients in an outpatient, behavioral therapy–oriented setting. Around the same time, we conducted a controlled matched-pairs study in a psychodynamic setting involving inpatient psychosomatic rehabilitation. In this study, one of the two groups received EMDR therapy in addition to the standard treatment (Hase et al., 2015). By the end of treatment, both studies showed a significant decrease in the severity of depression. During EMDR therapy, the processing of depression-related memory material was essential for treatment. Hofmann et al. (2014) showed that in the EMDR therapy group, the number of complete remissions of depressive episodes was approximately twice as high as it was in the group that received only the standard treatment. Additionally, Hase et al. (2015) demonstrated the lasting results of EMDR treatment with the finding that this group reported an increased ability to work compared to the second group at a 1-year follow-up.

In 2009, a European research association, the European Depression EMDR Network (EDEN), was initiated to further study depression and EMDR therapy. EDEN set the goal to reassess the data from the controlled studies in a randomized multicenter study. Additionally, this group of experienced clinicians and researchers continued to discuss the possibility of developing a treatment plan. In 2011, an internet-based database for randomization and collection of data was established under the direction of the University of Turin. Out of the original plan for seven treatment centers in three European countries, only three centers in Spain, Italy, and Germany became active. While the centers in Spain and Italy compared cognitive behavioral therapy (CBT) with EMDR, the German center primarily investigated the previous design, that is, standard treatment (pharmacotherapy with psychodynamic therapy) alone versus standard treatment plus processing of memories with EMDR therapy, but now under randomized, controlled conditions.

The data generated in the German center showed that even under randomized, controlled conditions, EMDR therapy had a statistically significant advantage over the standard treatment in terms of a reduction of depression scores at the end of treatment (Beck Depression Inventory, Second Edition [BDI-II]) and in terms of complete remissions (Hase et al., 2018). Once again, the number of complete remissions in the group that received EMDR was about double that of the standard treatment group.

The results of the Italian and Spanish centers require separate consideration. Since these patients received either CBT or EMDR as their standard treatments, the two approaches were compared directly. The size of the study corresponded to an equivalence study (a noninferiority study) to show whether a new treatment is no worse than a proven treatment to which it is being compared. The results showed that EMDR was as effective as the established procedure (i.e., CBT) in terms of the reduction of the severity of depression (BDI-II). However, the progression of the change over time is interesting and requires closer consideration. In the study, seven measurement times were defined and evaluated using the BDI-II. First, a baseline measurement was taken. The next measurement took place after 2 weeks, and then there were additional measurements after every four sessions. In addition to the measurement at the end of the intervention, there was an additional follow-up after 6 months. As part of the treatment, both groups received a phase of preparation and stabilization before the specific interventions began. In the EMDR group, this intervention was the processing of relevant memories according to the study protocol of the EDEN study. Figure 2.1 provides the change over time.

Here it becomes clear that the change in BDI-II in the preparation and stabilization phase develops similarly in both groups. With the beginning of the specific intervention—for the EMDR group, the processing of memories—the BDI-II drops more markedly in the EMDR group. This difference between both therapy approaches is the most significant in the study ($p < .001$). In this variance, one sees the difference between the symptom-oriented

Chapter 2 The EMDR Protocol for the Treatment of Depression   41

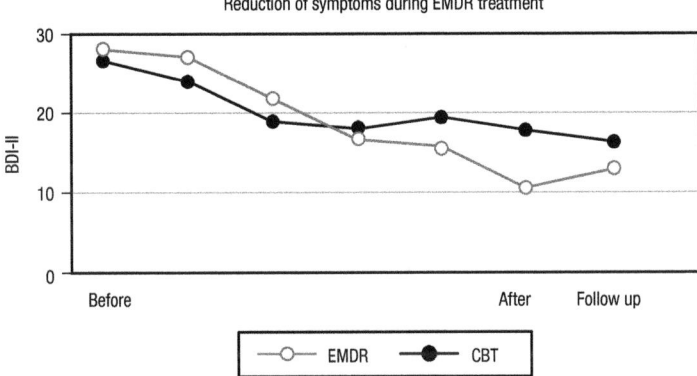

FIGURE 2.1. Progression of the severity of depression in the comparative study of EMDR therapy versus cognitive behavioral therapy (CBT).

Source: Data from Ostacoli, L., Carletto, S., Cavallo, M., Baldomir-Gago, P., Di Lorenzo, G., Fernandez, I., Hase, M., Justo-Alonso, A., Lehnung, M., Migliaretti, G., Oliva, F., Pagani, M., Recarey-Eiris, S., Torta, R., Tumani, V., Gonzalez-Vazquez, A. I., & Hofmann, A. (2018). Comparison of eye movement desensitization reprocessing and cognitive behavioral therapy as adjunctive treatments for recurrent depression: The European Depression EMDR Network (EDEN) randomized controlled trial. *Frontiers in Psychology, 9*, 74. https://doi.org/10.3389/fpsyg.2018.00074

intervention in CBT and the processing of pathogenic memories in EMDR that is aimed at the basis for the disorder.

The review by Malandrone et al. (2019) of the treatment of depression with EMDR therapy investigated six randomized controlled clinical trials (RCTs) and five controlled studies. Due to the activity of the EDEN network, results showed that the quality of the studies was improving and the data suggested that EMDR therapy is at least as effective in the treatment of depressive disorders as other psychotherapy approaches (equivalence). A new meta-analysis showed that EMDR has reduced the symptoms of depression at the end of treatment better than the control groups—including CBT (Yan et al., 2021).

The EDEN study manual, which was used in these studies and that we later called the DeprEnd Protocol, contains a treatment plan for the treatment of depressive patients with EMDR that is supported by scientific evidence. We will now present an overview of the DeprEnd treatment manual.

THE DeprEnd PROTOCOL

First, we present some important considerations. A *protocol* in EMDR therapy is a treatment plan that structures and prioritizes the order of treatment and is directed toward the processing of the distressing memories that cause the disorder. These memories include individual incidents as well as memory networks. It should be noted that the material presents the therapist with options for a range of EMDR procedures for working on the unprocessed memories. Even if one chooses the classic procedure for the reprocessing phases (Phases 4–6), other EMDR techniques can still be used, such as techniques with reduced associativity such as EMD or The Method of Constant Installation of Present Orientation and Safety (CIPOS), an EMDR-derived technique.

The DeprEnd Protocol that is used in EMDR therapy has eight phases. This means that in every protocol, Phase 1/History Taking, and Phase 2/Preparation and Stabilization, are included. Phase 1/History Taking informs therapists so that they can create a treatment plan with patients.

PHASE 1/HISTORY TAKING WHEN WORKING WITH DEPRESSIVE PATIENTS

There are some principles in handling depression that also retain their importance in EMDR therapy. These principles include: identify the memory networks that are to be processed later, assess the patient's resources, evaluate clinically the severity of depression, and check for suicidal tendencies. Although, McHugh et al. (2019) reported that the connection between reported suicidal ideation and actual suicide attempts seem to be weaker than had long been assumed, asking about suicidal ideation remains good practice.

Evaluating the severity of depression is clearly a clinical decision that can be supported through suitable tools such as the BDI-II or the Hamilton Depression Rating Scale (HDRS). Knowing the severity of depression is important in order to create the most successful treatment plan. When patients have a severe depression with low energy and restricted affect, reprocessing becomes difficult or even impossible. A case of this kind requires stabilization with antidepressant medication and careful Resource Activation. Our experience shows it is possible to combine EMDR therapy with antidepressant medication without complications. EMDR reprocessing is also possible after conducting electroconvulsive treatment (ECT), although the patient's capacity to tolerate reprocessing could be temporarily limited.

However, if a patient reports suicidal intentions with concrete plans and the inability to negotiate a no-harm agreement, it is necessary to protect the patient by taking appropriate antisuicidal precautions.

After evaluating the patient's resources, Phase 1 will continue with the development of a treatment plan, based on the Adaptive Information Processing (AIP) Model. Since the therapeutic relationship between patient and therapist also begins to develop in this phase, the therapist's sensitivity is required to avoid overwhelming the patient and to support the therapeutic relationship through appropriate measures. One of the diagnostic techniques that can be used in Phase 1 is the float back technique.

When developing a treatment plan, special attention should be devoted to symptoms and their underlying memory networks, as well as to memories that are particularly important for the etiology of depressive disorders such as:

- *Episode Triggers:* Memories of incidents that triggered a depressive episode (Episode Triggers). These are often experienced in a time frame of 4 to 8 weeks before the episode. Since the patient is generally fixated on their depressive existence that may have already persisted for months, this requires active questioning.
- *Intrusive Thoughts:* Stressful memories that lead to intrusive thoughts (active memory networks). These can be of a traumatic or non-traumatic nature. Special attention is given to memories of distressing experiences during early development (Teicher et al., 2018).
- *Dysfunctional Beliefs:* These manifest in the form of intrusive maladaptive thoughts like *I am worthless*. These cognitive intrusions generally indicate an early memory network of incidents. The childhood memories it contains are not always accessible, thus it is

Chapter 2   The EMDR Protocol for the Treatment of Depression   43

important to ask about *proof memories* or present memories that the patient uses as proof that the belief is true.
- *Persisting Present Triggers:* For material connected to past Episode Triggers or dysfunctional beliefs.
- *Evolving Adaptive Perceptions:* These are to address potential future challenges regarding past Episode Triggers or dysfunctional beliefs.
- *Depressive or Suicidal States:* Memories of being *depressive* or *suicidal*.

It is helpful to use a graphic tool to collect this information, such as the Symptom Event Map (Hofmann et al., 2016a, 2016b). This strategy makes it easier to plan the treatment.

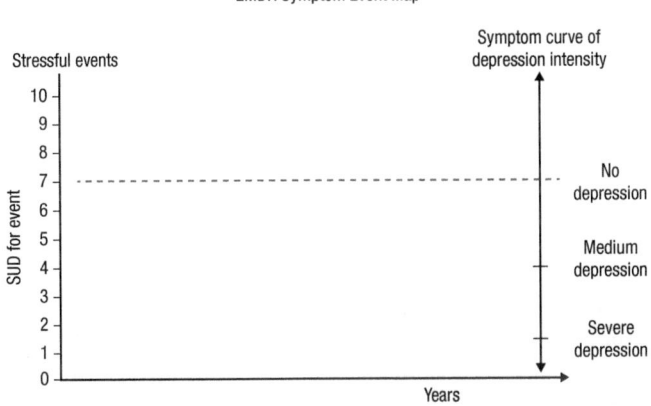

FIGURE 2.2. Symptom Event Map: On the timeline, when drawing the first map, the strength of symptoms is given as a curve (right-side scale/symptom curve). Connected with this is the second map (left-side scale) with the distressing memories that are recorded with their SUD on the timeline. The maps are different, but the combination allows the identification of depressive Episode Triggers.

SUD, Subjective Units of Disturbance.

Figure 2.2 shows the empty Symptom Event Map. First, to fill it out, patients are asked to list the depressive episodes that they experienced, including the present episode. These episodes are then listed and documented on the timeline of the map using the scale on the *x*-axis. Then, the distressing life experiences are documented in the same timeline using the Subjective Units of Disturbance (SUD) scale results on the *y*-axis. Seeing the results of their mood/degree of distress as a line on the map allows therapists and patients to recognize the relationship between distressing life experiences and changes in mood. Most important are the stressful incidents that have a temporal connection to the beginning of an episode; this is a constellation we call *Episode Triggers*.

In Figure 2.3, a male patient diagnosed with a major depressive episode came in for treatment. He separated from his partner 6 months earlier and reported a SUD of 10 for the event. Two years prior to that, he reported a medium depressive episode. Before this earlier episode began, he suffered from bullying and humiliation at his workplace. He then changed his job and recovered well from the depressive episode. (For a more detailed explanation of the Symptom Event Map, see Chapter 14.)

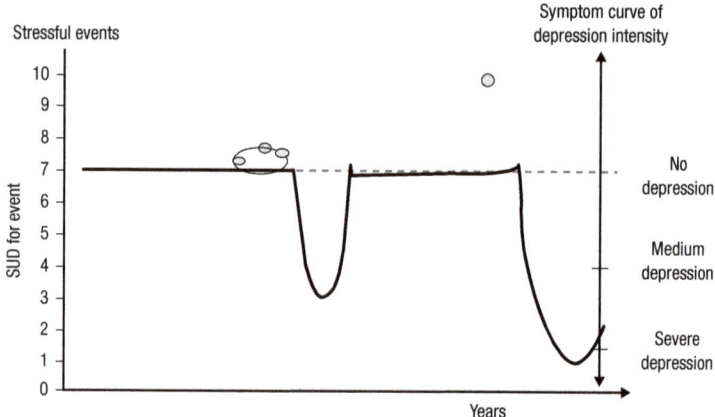

FIGURE 2.3. Symptom Event Map of a patient who came in with a major depressive episode. SUD, Subjective Units of Disturbance.

PHASE 2/PREPARATION AND STABILIZATION

Phase 2 always comes before working on pathogenic memories. In Phase 2 of patients' preparations, they receive a thorough explanation of their disorder, their suggested treatment plan, and EMDR therapy. The need for stabilization is dependent on the individual and will become apparent in the course of the first few sessions or occasionally over the course of the therapy. It is important to pay special attention to attachment-related traumas or experiences, such as early hospitalizations as a child and so on, because these can indicate an increased need for stabilization in terms of attachment. A lack of a foundation in attachment always means a complication in treatment. When this is the case, the therapeutic relationship requires special attention and stabilization, as it is essential to be prepared to prevent potential attachment-related crises over the course of treatment.

PHASES 3 TO 8: MEMORY WORK WITH PATHOGENIC MEMORIES

A typical EMDR treatment plan for treating depression contains the following memory-targeting sequence for EMDR reprocessing:

A. Processing of Episode Triggers

Incidents that initiated the beginning of an episode (Episode Triggers) are the first focus of EMDR therapy. These memories typically occur 4 to 8 weeks before the beginning of a depressive episode. Active questioning is required to identify these memories. Also, it is important to note how intrusive the memory is, as it is an important criterion. The memories are not always easy to identify, especially if the patient is still in the depressive episode, as their depressive symptoms have a large influence over their current experience. In this case, one begins with the trigger for the current episode and then expands to other Episode Triggers. Some Episode Triggers are not singular events, but clusters of events (like bullying in the workplace). In any case, it often works best if all emotionally charged events are mapped, specifically the first, the worst, and the last events, before the individual events of the cluster are processed.

If the current depressive episode has subsided, it is customary to begin with the trigger for the worst episode, and then expand the treatment to other Episode Triggers depending on the case. If the patient is suffering from chronic depression (episode has lasted for more than 2 years), it makes sense to work with events that cause the worsening of their mood.

Likewise, memories of traumatic or non-traumatic life events are reprocessed if these are distressing to the patient in an intrusive way. Even if these intrusive memories may not be Episode Triggers, such intrusions can be a sign of posttraumatic stress disorder (PTSD) or partial PTSD. Getting these intrusions addressed can relieve the distress of patients and is important in the treatment.

B. Processing of Negative Belief Systems

Depressive patients overwhelmingly report having dysfunctional belief systems. These thoughts that invade their consciousness can be understood as symptoms of a triggered memory network that are similar to the *negative cognitions* that are familiar to us from classical EMDR memory work. If the memory work with the Episode Trigger was successful and contributed to the patient's stabilization, proceed to work on the belief system, if this is supported by the patient's symptoms. Frequently, after patients process the Episode Triggers, the belief system becomes more prominent and for this reason, this change in focus is reasonable.

The task here is to search for dysfunctional beliefs and to create a hierarchy in terms of distress. In our experience, dysfunctional beliefs predominantly can be traced back to childhood memories that continue to be validated later by current experience when the memory work is triggered. The underlying memories are more difficult to access, especially at the beginning of treatment. It is easier to access the current realization of the material that the patient experiences during triggering. Since these memories continue to *prove* the validity of the dysfunctional belief, as it were, we call them *proof memories*, following de Jongh et al. (2010). Most distressing beliefs can be used as a starting point for exploring the underlying memory networks. You can also use techniques such as the affect bridge here as a diagnostic tool. If early charged memories are found, these can be organized in clusters according to the dysfunctional beliefs. Here, the cluster strategy is useful in processing. The workflow for the memory work in the belief system is as follows:

- Identify proof memories.
- Find other important, highly charged connected memories (like touchstone memories).
- Check and reprocess other proof memories and other highly charged memories from the network behind the belief system.
- Identify and process triggers for the beliefs identified at the beginning.
- Work with the patient's projections of the future or the future template for the identified beliefs.

C. Triggers and Future Work for Episode Triggers

After memory work with the belief system, continue with the following memories:

1. Identify triggers for memories in group A and reprocess as necessary.
2. Work with the patient's projections of the future or the future template for memories in group A. Depending on the clinical situation, these triggers, as well as the future projections, can also be processed after processing the Episode Triggers.

D. Processing of Depressive and Suicidal States

If working with the material from A to C leads to a stabilization of the patient, memories of the experience of their depressive symptoms—the feeling of *being* depressed or *being* suicidal—can be identified and reprocessed. In many cases, these somatic memories are overlooked so it is important to understand that experiencing depressive symptoms or suicidal tendencies can lead to an unprocessed memory due to the high degree of distress associated with this experience. When these symptoms have persisted for a while or there have been repeated suicidal thoughts, they can create a memory in patients of these depressive or suicidal thoughts and feelings. We have chosen the term *state* to designate this interesting phenomenon. This term is fundamentally different from the term *ego states*. The order of processing usually begins with the Depressive State and proceeds, if necessary, to the Suicidal State. If there is not one but several memories that can be identified, a cluster strategy should be considered (focusing on the earliest, worst, and most current memories—in this sequence).

1. Memories of depressive symptoms
2. Memories of suicidal tendencies

Processing a Suicidal State should only be performed after the patient has experienced the following: relief from their symptoms through their previous memory work; cessation of active suicidal tendencies; a strong therapeutic relationship; and distress from these states occurring due to their previous experience of suicidal tendencies or anxiety concerning their possible reappearance.

E. Relapse Prevention

After being treated with one or several of the steps of the EMDR depression protocol, most depressive patients usually come out of the current depressive episode. However, this is not the full comprehensive treatment for depression because many pathogenic memories or triggers may be left and are a risk factor for depressive relapse. In the relapse prevention aspect of our depression protocol, we try to identify and remove as many of those risk factors for future relapse as possible. Our studies show that this may be very effective in reducing future relapses in depressive patients.

USE DIFFERENT STRATEGIES FOR STRUCTURING REPROCESSING ACCORDING TO THE CLINICAL SITUATION

As mentioned, patients' symptoms can suggest a change in the ordering of targeting. If patients are primarily suffering from dysfunctional beliefs and other aspects of their memory (e.g., Episode Triggers) are not intrusive, then one may consider early memory work with patients' belief systems. As discussed under B. Processing of Negative Belief Systems, using the AIP Model may access the network of memories associated with the belief. However, be alert to the fact that underlying material from childhood may not yet be accessible, especially when this is attempted early in treatment and patients are seriously depressed. In such cases, it is worth starting by processing the proof memories, as patients can access these proofs more easily and often are already talking about them. The clinical effect of processing this *symptomatic* material is limited, but it can nonetheless provide patients with selective relief. After processing several proof memories, accessing the underlying memory network becomes more possible in some cases.

In principle, we can divide depressive patients into four groups, with each group benefitting from a different focusing strategy:

- *Depression Largely in Remission:* This first group consists of patients whose symptoms have by and large remitted, and for whom the depressive episode is nearly or already over. Here, focus first on the Episode Trigger for the worst episode. After this, additional Episode Triggers and other intrusive memories can be processed. Subsequently, processing continues in the order described previously.
- *Active Depression:* This second group is made up of patients who are actively in a depressive episode. Here, it is helpful to consider strengthening resources in order to mitigate their experience of depression. The order of processing here should begin with the trigger for the current episode, since patients are still very much fixated on their current experiences. After this, memory work can be extended to other Episode Triggers and other intrusive memories. If memory work is possible with patients' belief systems, reprocessing is continued in the order described previously.
- *Chronic Depression:* Patients who suffer from chronic depression (the depressive episode lasts for more than 2 years) require more stabilization through Resource Activation at the beginning of treatment. Identifying an Episode Trigger is often not possible due to the long duration of the episode and patients' strong fixation on the experience of their symptoms. However, depressive symptoms are not constant during the episode. One can identify fluctuations in their depression. When patients' moods worsen, it is worthwhile to search for current incidents that preceded the changes in mood. These are often situations involving a social interaction, for example, criticism or demands in their social environment that patients experience as overwhelming. This provides the opportunity to focus on this material, although the intensity of the chosen technique should not overwhelm patients. In memory work with patients' belief systems, it is often only possible to start reprocessing with proof memories at the beginning. Only after their depression has gotten better is it possible to access early memory networks for some patients. Here, one sees the usefulness of an *inverted* procedure, which Hofmann (2009) uses in his *Inverted Standard Protocol for Unstable Complex Post-Traumatic Stress Disorder,* and the EMDR stabilization techniques of Korn and Leeds (2002) and Hase (2021).
- *Chronic Depression and Complex PTSD/Other Severe Trauma-Related Disorders:* The comorbidity of chronic depression with complex PTSD or other severe trauma-related disorders is one of the greatest clinical challenges. Peritraumatic dissociation, defined as a complex array of reactions at the time of the trauma that include depersonalization, derealization, dissociative amnesia, out-of-body experiences, emotional numbness, and altered time perception that is frequently a part of the memory network, is often active in many unprocessed memories and can have an important influence on patients' conditions. This can contribute to a feeling of numbness, that may be confused with a symptom of severe depression. Often, the difference can be seen only in the course of a longer treatment after extensive processing of material. For these patients, often reprocessing the extensive belief systems is necessary. For patients who are

more stable in their everyday life, using the *Standard EMDR Protocol* is possible if the material initially is carefully selected and a graduated approach regarding the affect intensity of memory processing is used. For more unstable patients, proceeding by using the *Inverted EMDR Standard Protocol*, which starts with present stressors and moves on to more stressful memories in the past, makes sense. In any case, it is important to adapt the treatment plan to the current needs of the patient.

CLINICAL EXPERIENCE AND EXAMPLE CASES

There are several significant things we have learned from treating depressive patients. The first is that therapists need to be patient. The reward for therapists' patience is that treating patients with EMDR therapy leads to a more collaborative experience and less friction. An additional thing we have learned is that the positive cognition is available to the patient as a resource for later situations after the processing of the distressing material. The report from a patient who said, "*Earlier I would have gotten depressed again when I got news that my aunt is sick with cancer again, but now the statement 'I can handle this' is there!*" is an affirming experience, even for therapists.

When diagnosing and selecting material in conjunction with patients, the therapists' sensitivity is crucial. If therapists are treating patients with comorbid depression and PSTD or complex PTSD, a rigid treatment structure is not conducive to patients' needs. Rather, it will be necessary to move back and forth between the patients' need for stabilization versus processing maladaptive material. Moving forward includes assessing patients' distress, the intrusive memory networks, and patients' ability to process their material. It is important to assess if memories from their earlier life are accessible. Often, the treatment plan will use the *Inverted Standard EMDR Protocol*. Here are some examples to illustrate these issues.

Case Study 2.1

ADULT FEMALE WITH PERSISTENT DEPRESSIVE EPISODE

This 72-year-old retired female patient was in an outpatient day program, funded by her public health insurance, for her severe depression. The patient could not be convinced to receive inpatient treatment, and outpatient psychotherapy had not occurred. She reported that she had been helpless in her apartment for 24 hours after a stroke until her daughter noticed and called emergency services. Due to the stroke, she could not move her right arm and right leg and had been unable to get help for herself.

After an initial inpatient hospitalization, she went for rehabilitation and a psychotherapy program. Here, she was frightened by her physician when he said she would be dead within a year if she did not lose some weight. After this incident, her outlook changed dramatically. She had severe anxiety and became reclusive. She frequently called emergency services because she worried that she would have another stroke or that her blood pressure was too high. Her blood pressure was also difficult to regulate via medication. She felt very uncomfortable in her new apartment to which she had moved shortly before the stroke. She fought for a long time to get this apartment and now she described it as a dark cave and she would have preferred to move back into her old apartment. Unfortunately, this was not possible. She was depressed, nothing could make her happy, and she had no energy. This was in contrast to the time when she was first discharged from the hospital and went into a rehabilitation facility; then, she had some hope. She learned how to walk and speak again.

Based on the patient's description, I (M.H.) assumed that the experience of lying helplessly in the apartment was a quasitraumatic experience for her and that treatment using EMDR therapy would be helpful. After excellent rehabilitative care, the patient's neurological deficiencies were few. There remained a small weakness in the right arm and occasional subtle impairment in speech production. Otherwise, it seemed the patient would be able to cope with the stress of treatment. Further contraindications could not be determined during the diagnostic phase. Due to her age, her history taking included asking about war experiences. She denied any trauma during the war or since. After establishing the safe place, including bilateral eye movements, the first EMDR session took place. The patient chose to focus on the memory "The neurologist told me that I will die if I do not lose weight." It became clear that this was the Episode Trigger. We processed the memory in one session. Afterward, there was a marked improvement in the patient's mood and motivation. A week later, the memory of "lying helpless in the apartment" was brought into focus as another intrusive memory and reprocessed.

After 6 weeks of full-day rehabilitation with two EMDR memory processing sessions focusing on the Episode Trigger and another active memory network, the patient had improved markedly. Her depression and anxiety had decreased, and that was represented in the diagnostic tests. She now felt comfortable in her new apartment and saw it as bright and friendly. She made new social contacts and continued her activities outside of rehab. Her frequent calls to emergency services ended. She also contacted her primary care physician less frequently. After 12 months, her primary care physician reported that his patient now actually came in for follow-ups too little, as had been her practice before.

The dysfunctional beliefs, that were to some extent recognizable and resembled those of many "war babies" were well compensated and did not produce any classic symptoms. At this point, she had cleared the presenting problem and could be discharged from treatment.

Case Study 2.2

ADULT MALE WITH COMORBIDITY OF DEPRESSION AND PTSD

I (M.H.) met my 48-year-old male patient shortly before the end of his treatment for a depressive episode. When it was discovered later that he had psychological trauma in his history, he was sent to me for treatment. Treatment began 3 months after he was released from inpatient care. The patient presented with depressive and *traumatic-related symptoms. The trauma symptoms included intrusive thoughts, hypervigilance, and avoidance that began in his workplace.*

The patient was born in South Africa to a family of English descent. At the same time, the family's social situation was to some extent precarious. His mother had lost a child before the patient was born. This could have possibly affected his early-childhood attachment. His hot-tempered father continuously instilled fear in him. His progress in school was impeded by a stutter and unrecognized dyslexia. As a result of his teachers' sternness, he developed a stomach ulcer. His peer group at school rejected him. To some extent, he was able to compensate for this through active participation in youth groups at his church. With the diagnosis of his learning disability and appropriate support, he got better, and the patient was able to finish school and receive vocational training. Retrospectively, it can be assumed that there were already unrecognized depressive episodes in adolescence.

When he was 20, the patient was conscripted for military service. During the war in Angola, the patient experienced traumatization that led to the development of PTSD, as could be seen retrospectively. These symptoms "disappeared," probably as his social isolation, and not being accepted in society, became more dominant. The patient later emigrated to Europe to live with the woman who would become his wife. In Europe, he went through training to become a social worker and worked later in an institute for residential youth services. His first marriage failed and this triggered his first depressive episode. At the time, the patient did not seek treatment. The patient then entered another marriage. This marriage has remained stable until today. He is the father of a daughter.

In May 2015, he was attacked with a knife by an adolescent resident who was in a state of agitation. This led to the development of PTSD symptoms that were initially recorded but not treated. In November 2015, the ensuing difficulties at work contributed to the development of a severe depressive episode, that led to an inpatient treatment; however, no trauma-specific treatment was performed and the symptoms persisted. The patient was discharged as fully recovered and insurance refused to cover any further costs. As the patient continued to be unable to work, he was hospitalized again in the summer of 2016, at the expense of his pension insurance plan. This hospitalization produced no substantial success due to the complexity and severity of his case, but it did lead the patient to outpatient treatment.

In outpatient treatment, I began to understand the complex nature of this patient's disorder after several history-taking sessions. The patient suffered from typical PTSD symptoms related to the recent event at work, nightmares related to his traumatization while at war, and a moderate depression (BDI-II: 22), that had persisted for 18 months. He was being stabilized with escitalopram. The diagnostic work and his psychoeducation regarding EMDR therapy led to a supportive therapeutic relationship. Unfortunately, the beginning of therapy was delayed by disputes about whose responsibility it was for covering the costs of treatment, with the result that by the time we started our work together, he had a chronic depression.

When we began therapy, the patient's symptoms of PTSD were clear. For this reason, after processing a smaller memory to introduce the patient to EMDR, I began with the processing of material related to the traumatization at the workplace, the Episode Trigger. It was possible to process the material in 6 sessions. In the session with this memory, I used the EMDR-CIPOS technique to titrate the experience so he could experience some relief. The intrusions related to this incident and the hypervigilance decreased.

After this, I began to process the worsening of his mood by looking for triggers of small aggravations of his depressive mood. Next, we mainly dealt with disputes with health insurers. Accompanied by a competent attorney, the patient began his long road to receiving retraining. This led to an activation of the patient's dysfunctional beliefs such as "I don't deserve it" and "I am a loser." Now, we were able to get access to the triggering memory networks from childhood via proof memories and to focus on touchstone memories (DeprEnd Group B). Also, we made the first attempt at reaching these difficult memories with EMDR-CIPOS and/or EMD (Shapiro, 2018). Despite the difficulty of working through these memories, this led to a slow improvement of his mood. Along with processing the memories, I was also repeatedly able to install the position of power and attachment-related resource installation/Instant Resource Installation (IRI). Then, we focused on the processing of triggers for his beliefs (DeprEnd Group B4) and the installation of a future template for the triggers (DeprEnd Group B5).

Working with his belief system took about 20 sessions. With his improved mood, the patient began receiving professional retraining. As he began to participate in life more actively, triggers concerning his traumatization in the workplace arose, and we worked on this material (DeprEnd Group C1). After processing the triggers, a future template (Shapiro, 2018) was installed in each case (DepreEnd Group C2). Subsequently, memories about his Depressive State were processed (DeprEnd Group D1). By now, the patient had finished his retraining and had begun work. His mood had stabilized significantly. There was still therapeutic work on his war traumatization to do, but he had few symptoms there and we would see if this material provoked symptoms in the future. In total, 40 sessions of EMDR therapy had been completed by this point.

This treatment follows the guidelines of the DeprEnd Protocol, however, it also shows the flexibility needed by a perceptive therapist to repeatedly deviate from it in response to the patient's complex symptoms.

REFERENCES

de Jongh, A., ten Broeke, E., & Meijer, S. (2010). Two method approach: A case conceptualization model in the context of EMDR. *Journal of EMDR Practice and Research*, 4(1), 12–21. https://doi.org/10.1891/1933-3196.4.1.12

Hase, M. (2021). Instant resource installation and extensive resource installation—Two novel techniques for resource installation in EMDR therapy—Theory, description and case report. *European Journal of Trauma & Dissociation*, 5(4). https://doi.org/10.1016/j.ejtd.2021.100224

Hase, M., Balmaceda, U. M., Hase, A., Lehnung, M., Tumani, V., Huchzermeier, C., & Hofmann, A. (2015). Eye movement desensitization and reprocessing (EMDR) therapy in the treatment of depression: A matched pairs study in an inpatient setting. *Brain and Behavior*, *5*(6), e00342. https://doi.org/10.1002/brb3.342

Hase, M., Plagge, J., Hase, A., Braas, R., Ostacoli, L., Hofmann, A., & Huchzermeier, C. (2018). Eye movement desensitization and reprocessing versus treatment as usual in the treatment of depression: A randomized-controlled trial. *Frontiers in Psychology*, *14*(9), 1384. https://doi.org/10.3389/fpsyg.2018.01384

Hofmann, A. (2009). The Inverted EMDR Standard Protocol for unstable complex posttraumatic stress disorder. In M. Luber (Ed.), *Eye movement desensitization and reprocessing: EMDR scripted protocols. Special populations* (pp. 313–328). Springer Publishing Company.

Hofmann, A., Hilgers, A., Lehnung, M., Liebermann, P., Ostacoli, L., Schneider, W., & Hase, M. (2014). Eye movement desensitization and reprocessing (EMDR) as an adjunctive treatment in depression: A controlled study. *Journal of EMDR Practice and Research*, *8*(3), 103–112. https://doi.org/10.1891/1933-3196.8.3.103

Hofmann, A., Hase, M., Liebermann, P., Ostacoli, L., Lehnung, M., Ebner, F., Rost, C., Luber, M. & Tumani, V. (2016a). DeprEnd® – EMDR therapy protocol for the treatment of depressive disorders. In M. Luber (Ed.), *EMDR therapy scripted protocols and summary sheets: Treating anxiety, obsessive-compulsive, and mood-related conditions* (pp. 289–323). Springer Publishing Company.

Hofmann, A., Hase, M., Liebermann, P., Ostacoli, L., Lehnung, M., Ebner, F., Rost, C., Luber, M., & Tumani, V. (2016b). An EMDR protocol for the treatment of depression. In M. Luber (Ed.), *EMDR scripted protocols: Treating anxiety, obsessive-compulsive, and mood-related conditions* (pp. 290–311). Springer Publishing Company.

Korn, D. L., & Leeds, A. M. (2002). Preliminary evidence of efficacy for EMDR Resource Development and Installation in the stabilization phase of treatment of complex posttraumatic stress disorder. *Journal of Clinical Psychology*, *58*(12), 1465–1487. https://doi.org/10.1002/jclp.10099

Malandrone, F., Carletto, S., Hase, M., Hofmann, A., & Ostacoli, L. (2019). A brief narrative summary of randomized controlled trials investigating EMDR treatment of patients with depression. *Journal of EMDR Practice and Research*, *13*(4), 302–306. https://doi.org/10.1891/1933-3196.13.4.302

McHugh, C. M., Corderoy, A., Ryan, C. J., Hickie, I. B., & Large, M. M. (2019). Association between suicidal ideation and suicide: Meta-analyses of odds ratios, sensitivity, specificity and positive predictive value. *BJPsych Open*, *5*(2), E18. https://doi.org/10.1192/bjo.2018.88

Teicher, M. H., Anderson, C. M., Ohashi, K., Khan, A., McGreenery, C. E., Bolger, E. A., Rohan, M. L., & Vitaliano, G. D. (2018). Differential effects of childhood neglect and abuse during sensitive exposure periods on male and female hippocampus. *NeuroImage*, *169*, 443–452. https://doi.org/10.1016/j.neuroimage.2017.12.055

Yan, S., Shan, Y., Zhong, S., Miao, H., Luo, Y., Ran, H., & Jia, Y. (2021). The effectiveness of eye movement desensitization and reprocessing toward adults with major depressive disorder: A meta-analysis of randomized controlled trials. *Frontiers in Psychiatry*, *12*, 700458. https://doi.org/10.3389/fpsyt.2021.700458

3

Preparation and Stabilization in EMDR Therapy for Depressive Patients

Luca Ostacoli, Sara Carletto, Carmen Settanta, Lorena Giovinazzo, and Francesca Malandrone

INTRODUCTION

Many depressive patients come into psychotherapy treatment with little focus, decreased energy, and a loss of confidence in themselves. In this chapter, the authors focus on helping patients learn about their emotions, accept their protective emotions, and reconnect with their enriching emotions. They teach many different resources such as the container, paying attention to the five senses, breathing, and learning how to regulate vegetative systems. Also, they teach patients to stay within their window of tolerance and how to manage themselves when they are outside of it. In the stabilization section, the authors teach therapists to use many techniques in the service of self-regulation and self-care: the Self-Contact Technique, diaphragmatic breathing, grounding, aligning, glimpsing the *Hidden Heart: The Magic Query*, Hakomi's 3-Step Procedure, and the Triple Thanksgiving.

THE CORE OF DEPRESSION

Depression is one of the most common psychological disorders. According to the research criteria of the World Health Organization's (WHO) *International Classification of Diseases, Tenth Edition (ICD-10*; WHO, 1992), classification of mental disorders, depression is characterized by the following features:

1. Depressed mood, to a degree clearly unusual for the individual, most of the day, almost every day, essentially unaffected by circumstances, and persisting for at least 2 weeks

2. Interests and pleasure loss in activities that were normally enjoyable
3. Decreased drive or increased fatigue
4. Loss of self-confidence or self-esteem
5. Unfounded self-reproach or pronounced, inappropriate feelings of guilt
6. Recurrent thoughts of death or suicide, suicidal behavior
7. Complaints or evidence of decreased ability to think or concentrate, indecisiveness or indecision
8. Psychomotor agitation or inhibition
9. Sleep disturbances of any kind
10. Morning sickness
11. Loss of appetite or increased appetite with corresponding change in weight
12. Loss of libido

Exclusion criteria are:

1. The episode is not due to abuse of psychotic substances or to an organic mental disorder.
2. No manic or hypomanic symptoms are reported.

A limitation of this classification is the fact that many heterogeneous situations that also have different therapeutic indications fall under the diagnosis of major depressive disorder. From an affective point of view, the common element of depression seems to be the loss of the ability to love oneself, others, or life. The purpose of therapy should be to help people to gradually recover this connection. There can be different causes that lead to this reduction or loss of love in people's lives, such as the failure to mourn a loved one, an overwhelming difficulty that needs to be faced, or the inability to manage and overcome situations of profound complexity related to physical or mental illnesses. Whatever the causes of depression, as mentioned, a common factor is the reduction or loss of the ability to love with the first sign being the reduction of the ability to feel pleasure that generally precedes the onset of widespread sadness. The decrease in interest and motivation is also the element that makes it difficult for patients to improve their life quality. From the earliest stages of treatment, it is important to help patients understand that they have not really lost their ability to love but that their own internal balance system is protecting and keeping their affections hidden within. The feelings of connection are something sensitive and delicate compared to the difficulties of life that patients encounter and they await the opportunity to be able to express themselves again.

The entire course of therapy is a combination of practices to help people accept their emotions, even if they are difficult. The goals are to help patients have no fear of their emotions. This is done by helping them reconnect with themselves so that they can transform their interpretation of reality in a more constructive manner, and as a result, reopen the *blockages* that occurred after traumatic and stressful events so that they can discover new internal and external resources.

An important component is the encounter with the parts of one's own childhood to recognize them, accept them, and enable the resumption of their natural development. The great guide of this journey is nature itself. When we were born, nature assigned us the mission of living and helping others to live and provided us with powerful tools such as awareness, emotions, and relationships. By deeply understanding their value and learning to experience them, the road to freedom can reopen.

PREPARATION RESOURCES FROM NATURE: PROTECTIVE AND ENRICHING EMOTIONS

People suffering from depression very often misrecognize emotions as *symptoms* and avoid them. It is crucial to help them with psychoeducation to change their attitudes toward feelings and their bodily sensations.

Example of Psychoeducation for Emotions

Emotions are fundamental instruments that life has given us to guide us in the complexities of reality, overcoming difficulties, and living and having relationships. Too often the value of these emotions is misunderstood and is interpreted as *symptoms* that need to be eliminated. It is crucial to re-evaluate emotions as powerful, adaptive, natural processes (Berthoz et al., 2000; Flynn & Rudolph, 2014; Kranzler et al., 2016).

Everyone has their own way of perceiving and reacting to emotions that vary from one moment to the next. Sometimes we feel in tune with our feelings, other times we feel disoriented by suffering or maybe by pleasure; we push emotions away or we allow ourselves to be dragged around by them. When a painful experience is very intense, it can overwhelm us, leading to counterproductive defensive reactions. Other times, instead, we discover that we are able to face such experiences, even beyond our own personal expectations.

In order to understand the resources that our emotions hold, it is important to understand their nature and learn to experience them. Emotions can be divided into two main categories: not *negative* and *positive* ones but, instead, *protective* and *enriching emotions*.

Protective emotions are initially unpleasant because they help us recognize the potential damaging impact of events on us. Since they are uncomfortable, they are often erroneously considered *negative* emotions and therefore *to be pushed away*. It is fundamental to understand that they are really there to protect us. If we learn to pay attention to them, as we would do toward a loved one who comes to help us in a time of need, we would discover that their course is similar to going over a *hill*. Initially, our suffering grows, but once it reaches its peak, it diminishes and leaves us the resources needed to overcome the difficulty. This could be, for example, a sense of relief, confidence, clarity—whatever we need in that moment. They are like colors in the sense that there are only a few basic emotional *colors* that combine to create an infinite palette of emotional hues. These include anger, fear, sadness, and disgust. Like musical chords, emotions have different notes, but each moment has a *dominant* note. Each emotion offers an answer: For instance, anger helps us make our needs known; fear helps protect us from danger; disgust helps us keep our distance; and sadness, often misunderstood as a weakness, is the emotion of transformation that allows us to leave whatever cannot continue and transforms the qualities gleaned in the previous experience into a new context. If we learn to experience these emotions, they will allow us to exit the tunnel we have been in and get back into life.

Enriching emotions are more pleasant, if we are not afraid to experience them. They have many names and similar functions; for example, tenderness, affection, curiosity, pleasure, joy, recognition, and confidence. If we cultivate them every day, especially in the little things that we tend to take for granted, they help us to live the present moment to the fullest. Often, in order to feel fully the enriching emotions, we must first experience the protective emotions (Figure 3.1)! The risk behind the enriching emotions is to remain trapped in the pleasant moments by trying to relive them constantly. This leads to not being in the present moment and avoiding experiencing the riches of possibilities by devaluing whatever we think may interrupt these feelings. It is therefore imperative to learn how to savor them when they arrive, but also let them go. Only in this way will we be able to experience these emotions freely without becoming stuck.

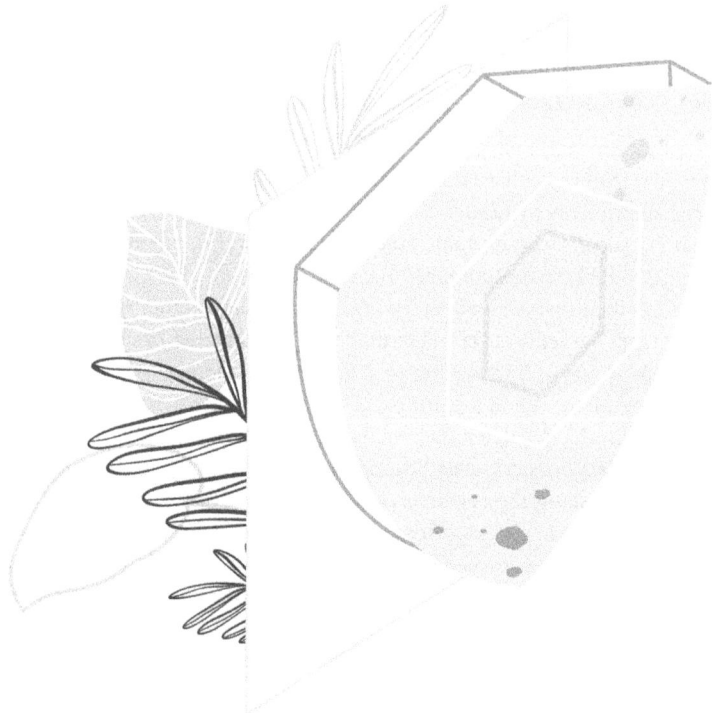

FIGURE 3.1. Enriching and protective emotions. The protective emotions are the shield behind which the enriching emotions can grow.

The emotions that allow us to access our resources are the authentic emotions; they arise throughout our lives to help us. The secondary emotions disguise the authentic emotions; for example, anger covering up sadness or fear, or sadness that camouflages anger, and so forth in all of the various combinations. How can we distinguish between authentic and secondary emotions? An important way is observing the effects they have on us and our relationships with others. The authentic emotions tend to be spontaneous with a sensation of newness; they blossom from within and are experienced throughout our bodies. Experiencing these emotions brings relief or greater clarity as we grow closer in our relationship with ourselves and with others. Repetitive thoughts tend to give rise to secondary emotions. They accumulate inside of us without giving us any relief; rather they grow and feed into our frustration and tend to push us away from others.

When we feel unpleasant emotions, the most important thing *not* to do is react impulsively and allow our emotions to drag us around, as this may result in our becoming aggressive and therefore counterproductive. Instead, it is important to establish a space that allows us to *observe* our emotions. Here, we can note where these emotions present themselves in our body by listening to and feeling the physical sensations of their manifestation and welcoming them with our breathing, for as long as we feel like, even if it is for a short moment. In this way, we create a space, even if just a little one, that allows us to *respond* instead of react, which is more helpful to us and for others. Authentic emotions manifest themselves in an area between the abdomen and the throat, usually in the chest or opening to the stomach. Secondary emotions, if you are able to pay attention to their physical sensations in the body, change rapidly into the authentic emotions described in the following.

Note: However, if we find ourselves in a life-threatening situation, we may have to respond quickly to the threat.

It is important to remember that emotions tend to evolve in waves that initially intensify, then weaken in intensity, while leaving behind resources. If we are facing particularly important life events, there will be many waves, with each wave bringing its part of relief when we learn to follow our own rhythms.

Regulating Volume of Emotions

When emotions are too intense, there are many ways to *regulate their volume*. Some useful suggestions are the following:

- *The Container:* We can effectively listen to or feel our emotions—at the same time in which we perceive them—only when we are inside our own window of tolerance. This can happen if the situation allows and if we indeed are paying attention to them. When these emotions are too intense and the moment is not right, we can imagine putting them into a *container*. In doing this, we actually visualize the emotions as they enter the container where they will be protected as objects of value, with the promise to return to them when possible. Our relationship with emotions is basically similar to the relationship of trust with children. If we actually go to children as soon as possible and take care of them, they will learn to put their trust in us and wait. If we do not attend to them, they learn not to pay attention to emotions and the next time we tell them to be patient, they will not do so and will continue to demand a response because of this lack of attention. It is important to build a relationship of trust with our emotions. If they are intense, it is better to postpone dealing with them, even if just for a short period of time, in order to choose when and how to do so. The choice renders us active participants and increases our ability to handle them when they catch us by surprise.
- *Be Friendly to Ourselves:* The first thing to do in dealing with emotion is to be as kind as possible to ourselves in the same way we would be with a loved one.
- *Posture:* Posture is very important. We can approach our emotions with greater strength if we feel the support we get from the ground or any surface that holds us up. This allows us to feel our core and this can give us a feeling of dignity.
- *Emotions Are Transient and We Are Greater Than They Are:* Sometimes our emotions surround us as if we were in a cloud, and make us lose sight of reality. It is important to remember that we are greater than any emotion, and that they are always transient—they come, wrap around us, and then recede.
- *Maintain Perception of the Here and Now Through the Five Senses:* We perceive the here and now through our five senses; for example, perceiving the points of contact that let us feel the support from the ground, the air against our skin, and the experience of our body as a whole. Emotional sensations make up only a small part of all our senses. It

could help to take a shower or incorporate activities that can open up our perception, including manual labor or taking a walk in nature.
- *Diaphragmatic Breathing:* Remember that thoracic/shallow breathing often brings more thoughts and anxiety, while diaphragmatic/deeper breathing is very useful to center us.
- *Movement:* Physical exercise can be very useful to re-access our perception of our bodies. When intense emotions present themselves, aerobic activity is particularly useful, such as walking, running, biking, or swimming as they assist in mobilizing energy and regulating our activation levels.
- *Sharing:* If possible, sharing with someone who knows how to listen without judging can be very useful. It is amazing how LISTENING to someone or to nature can be very helpful. By welcoming the positive qualities in others, we learn to change our perspective about our own qualities, thereby reducing the curtain of emotional fog that can confuse us.
- *Creative Expression:* As an alternative, emotions can be expressed creatively through writing, drawing, or through any other expressions of the experience we are living.

REGULATION OF AROUSAL AND PROCESSING: THE WINDOW OF TOLERANCE

Everything that happens in the body, both physiologically and psychologically, is mediated in its expression by the autonomic nervous system (Alvares et al., 2016; Kreibig, 2010). It is divided into two systems: sympathetic and parasympathetic (Figure 3.2). As in the Chinese Yin and Yang, with which there are many analogies, the parasympathetic function and the sympathetic function alternate throughout the day at many levels. For example, every time we breathe, when we inhale, we have a sympathetic response expressed which includes an increase in heart rate and pressure; every time we exhale, we have a parasympathetic response with a reduction in heart rate and pressure. The alternation of the sympathetic–parasympathetic symptoms does not only concern the heart but also all the organs of the body. We have a sympathetic response when we are awake during the day and a predisposition to a parasympathetic response in the night when we are asleep. In the autumn months, when the light is lower in the sky, and there is less activation, we have a greater parasympathetic activation, while in the summer months, there is a tendency to have a greater sympathetic activation, due to the light and the greater social stimuli. The balance of the sympathetic and parasympathetic systems regulates both physiological and relational functioning and the reaction to events (Mulkey & du Plessis, 2019; Porges, 2009).

One of the theories that can help to explain some of these important mechanisms is the Polyvagal Theory of Porges (Porges, 2001, 2009, 2011). Even if some important research questions regarding the theory are still not answered, especially regarding its controversial anatomical basis, the theory can be helpful clinically and explain some neurovegetative observations, at least until research will be able to better clarify the underlying neurobiological mechanisms.

In the Polyvagal Theory, three autonomic states are defined:

- *State of Security and Affiliation:* It takes place in safe relationships, no defense mechanisms are activated. This is characterized by the opening of sensory channels,

Chapter 3 Preparation and Stabilization in EMDR Therapy

receptiveness to the stimuli of the context and the possibility of empathy. An example could be a relationship with a dear person or a mother with her child.
- *Mobilization Defenses:* They take place when there is an event we have to face that includes fight or flight. There is predominantly sympathetic activation and limb involvement.
- *Immobilization Defenses:* They activate when we are facing an event we are not able to overcome by fight or flight. There is predominantly parasympathetic activation and limb deactivation with hypoarousal. An example is the simulated death of the mouse when it has been caught by the cat.

When there is a sympathetic–parasympathetic response that takes place in what Siegel (1999) defines as a *window of tolerance* (Figure 3.2), we are functioning well both physiologically and psychologically, we can experience emotions and relationships and think calmly about our thoughts. If, instead, the activation occurs outside the window of tolerance, we are out of balance (Corrigan et al., 2011; Ogden et al., 2006). See Figure 3.2.

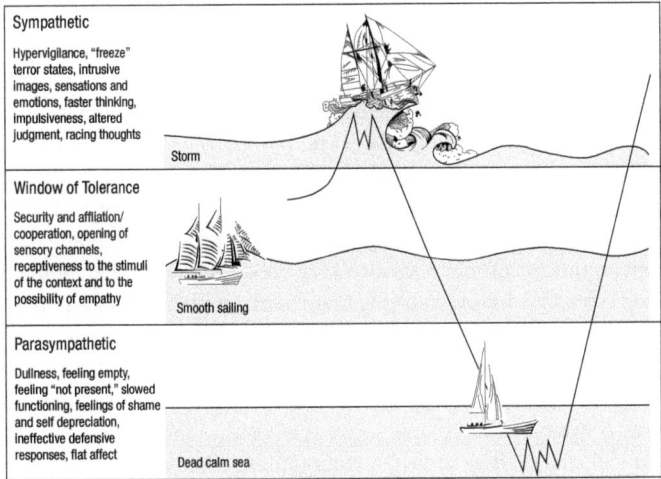

FIGURE 3.2. A graphic representation of the window of tolerance and the journey of life.

When the response is predominantly sympathetic, we have an increase in arousal thoughts and heart rate. It feels like we are in a state of alarm. Alternately, when we are in a predominantly parasympathetic state, we have a reduction in energy, mental blunting if not actual blocking out thoughts altogether or fainting. From a psychotherapeutic point of view, sympathetic activation is a state of hyperarousal defined as *Fight or Flight*, because the most frequent manifestations are those of fight or flight. However, it can also present as the Attachment Cry characterized by a request for help made directly to the attachment figure or by engaging in behavior requiring attention, or by Freezing which combines sympathetic and parasympathetic activation (Kozlowska et al., 2015; Ogden & Fisher, 2015; Porges, 2005; Roelofs, 2017).

When the parasympathetic system is activated, we are in a state of hypoarousal; the system involved is the *Rest or Digest*, systems that provide for the regulation of rest and digestion. It can, in fact, manifest itself through the gastrointestinal system with nausea that can lead to vomiting.

When the *Rest* part is activated, we feel a reduction in energy, blunted affect, drowsiness and lowering of pressure until fainting can occur; this can be defined as *Simulated Death*. It is an analogy to the defense that animals use when faced with a predator who is an overwhelming presence and cannot be opposed (Kozlowska et al., 2015; Minton et al., 2006; Ogden & Fisher, 2015).

In reality, these two systems are not contrasting but oscillating moment by moment: Like the seat of a swing, the more it is pushed upward on one side, the more it will tend to be high on the other; the greater the sympathetic activation, the more the parasympathetic one will be. When we talk about *hyper* or *hypo*, we refer to the center of gravity of this oscillation between the two states, in other words the mid-point of the oscillation. In fact, even in states of hyperactivation there will be parasympathetic symptoms such as blunting of affect, even to the freeze—which is a mixture of sympathetic hyperactivation and parasympathetic hyperactivation.

A surprising aspect that has been confirmed by neurobiological research is the fact that when we encounter an emotional experience, consisting of images, emotions, sensations, and thoughts, simply remaining in contact with them and staying within the window of tolerance, processing is spontaneously activated and effective (Braunstein et al., 2017; Guendelman et al., 2017; Ogden & Fisher, 2015; Sayers et al., 2015). Being in touch with our own emotions is the principle that unites mindfulness and eye movement desensitization and reprocessing (EMDR), in both cases the main force is to *stay present* as the participant observer, trusting the process!

To be able to process emotional states, it is necessary to be within the window of tolerance: Similar to a stereo, if the volume of emotions is too low to the point it sounds like noise, cognitive functions are reduced with a decrease in processing emotions This could happen when working on patients' trauma when they are in a hypoaroused state. When hyperarousal occurs, the excess of emotional *volume* makes the processing difficult and can be perceived as traumatizing itself, often resulting in negative impact also on the therapeutic alliance with patients. Patients' windows of tolerance also vary between one another. Some have a strong resilience and a very wide window, allowing them to maintain lucidity and the ability to manage, even when faced with difficult events. Others have a very narrow window of tolerance and get distressed even about small events.

One fundamental goal of therapy is to widen the window. If the window of tolerance is widened and resilience is increased, many events fall within the window of tolerance, reducing their emotional charge. It is, in fact, a common experience that, after having processed some traumas, other events are no longer perceived as disturbing (Ehlers et al., 2012; Iyadurai et al., 2019; Shapiro, 2014). The widening takes place by working on the upper limit of the window of tolerance. We could make a comparison with the sporting activity that is regulated by the same sympathetic–parasympathetic balance. An untrained person will have palpitations and be short of breath even for very limited exertion, but if they train progressively, they will increase their tolerance and will be able to withstand unthinkable levels of exertion compared to when they started. The same thing happens from an emotional point of view and is a basic tenet of many exposure techniques. The more a person is exposed to triggers at the upper limit of their window, the more they increase their resilience. The more they use avoidance strategies, the more they will be relieved in that moment because they move away from the stimulus; however, the more the window of tolerance is diminished, the less able patients are to face their reality. This is the genesis of most anxiety disorders where the main mechanism is, indeed, avoidance (Hofmann & Hay, 2018; Salters-Pedneault et al., 2004).

The very definition of trauma is subjective, linked not only to the scope of the event but also to the resilience of a person (Boals, 2018; Keshet et al., 2019; Weinberg & Gill, 2016).

Chapter 3 Preparation and Stabilization in EMDR Therapy

The greater the resilience, the less the events are perceived as traumatic, whereas when the window of tolerance is very narrow and consequently the resilience is very low, almost every event is perceived as traumatic.

It is important to be able to recognize when you are inside or outside the window of tolerance. To define that a person is outside of it, we cannot rely only on the intensity of the emotion, because emotions can sometimes be very intense, but we can be aware of what we are feeling and be balanced. To be outside the window is clinically defined by at least two out of three conditions:

1. When we are dominated by our emotional state and we lose control of our ability to think in a clear fashion
2. When we lose awareness to the point we cannot describe what is happening
3. When in this state, we lose our relational capacity and our empathic representation of the other (Corrigan et al., 2011; Ogden & Fisher, 2015), while the therapist feels the loss of connection with the person

Vice versa, when we are inside the window of tolerance, we are present in the here and now, with the potential to be aware of our feelings, emotions, and thoughts and can relate to others. To see if patients are in the window of tolerance, ask exploratory questions about their experience; when patients are able to describe their feelings, emotions, or thoughts, they are likely to be inside the window. Observing the physical sensations of emotions, the *felt sense*, described by E. T. Gendlin (1969), represents one of the main routes to being fully present in the *here and now* during the processing of emotions.

Another integrative modality is the somatic tracking of signs of hyperarousal, hypoarousal, and presence in the relationship (see sympathetic and parasympathetic somatic signs). One of therapists' fundamental tasks is to monitor where patients are concerning the window of tolerance and help them adjust their arousal according to the objectives of the work. It is more effective for patients to be in the middle of the window of tolerance while working on developing resources or discussing cognitive aspects of the issue(s).

In working on stressful life events, it is important to be in the medium high level of the window of tolerance, because if the activation is too low there is not enough energy to process the emotions connected to the event. Dealing with an event is like climbing a hill: On one side there are uncomfortable emotions, however, when going over and down the other side, activation not only can reduce but it can change the representation of the event and the resources that we need to adapt to reality may be more available to consciousness. However, energy is needed to climb that hill!

A simple way to distinguish sympathetic activation from parasympathetic is to ask whether that function could be useful in a fight. If the answer is affirmative, we are facing the sympathetic function of *Fight or Flight*, if it is not useful, there is the parasympathetic function of *Rest and Digest*. For example, during a fight, is it useful to have abundant salivation? No. In fact, the sympathetic response results in a reduction in secretions, and the parasympathetic activity increases. Is it useful to have intestinal peristalsis during a fight? No. In fact, sympathetic hyperarousal leads to constipation while parasympathetic hypoarousal tends to lead to diarrhea. On a digestive and metabolic level, we can see that during a fight, it is necessary to channel our energy into our reserves: The sympathetic response is *catabolic* because it tends to reduce glycogen reserves by mobilizing energy and increasing the presence of glucose in the blood. The parasympathetic response does the opposite and increases the deposit of glycogen into storage and reduces the catabolic response in favor of *anabolism*. Anabolism is a metabolic process that transforms simple substances into complex molecules and results in the repair of wounds and the storage of energy (Porges, 2011).

Autonomic regulation is not only of an emotional origin, but includes physical lifestyle activities such as diaphragmatic breathing, physical activity, nutrition, sleep hygiene, social relationships, and pleasure. These kinds of activities play a fundamental role in self-regulation; maintaining a good sympathetic–parasympathetic balance through them means helping to expand the window of tolerance both physically and emotionally.

Strong physical activity improves autonomic stabilization and could *cover up* unresolved trauma, similarly to antidepressant drugs (Rosenbaum et al., 2015). For example, if people stopped exercising because they had inflammation due to tendinitis or an accident, it could result in hyperarousal of the nervous system because of the decrease of endorphins, and they could have a reactivation of the traumatic aspect because exercise was no longer masking their symptoms. Physical activity can be utilized in psychotherapy as a protective role, especially for Depressive States characterized by hypoarousal (Phillips et al., 2003; Rebar et al., 2015; Rosenbaum et al., 2015).

Similarly, nutrition is important. If we take into account that the sympathetic response is mainly active during the day and is catabolic, meaning it translates the body reserves into energy, while the parasympathetic system is anabolic and tends to favor depositing energy during rest, it becomes clear how important an adequate breakfast in the morning can contribute to increasing our energy and mood, and a diet that focuses on eating more in the evening can have negative effects on sleep by overloading it with digesting at a time where the body needs to rest. Today, there are many studies that correlate the effect of nutrition on mood and on energy, and the importance of regulating them by taking into account autonomic rhythms (Lassale et al., 2019; Opie et al., 2015; Stevenson, 2017).

Another element that has a central role in autonomic regulation is breathing (Jerath et al., 2015), and due to its importance, there is a special section in this chapter dedicated to the use of breath in psychotherapeutic work.

Normally, alternating sympathetic and parasympathetic arousal results in a balance (Porges, 2009). When a stressful stimulus appears, the sympathetic reaction prevails until the stimulus subsides; that is, if the stressful event is something the person can manage actively (Figure 3.3). Its role is to support mobilizing actions and inhibit the functioning

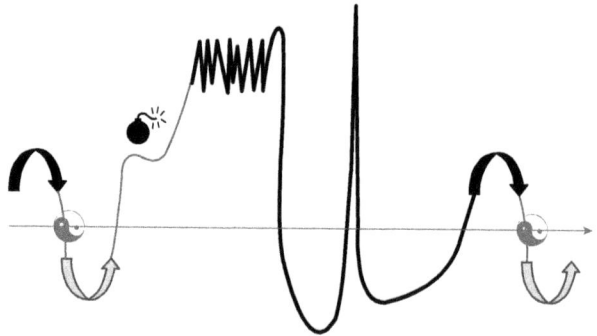

FIGURE 3.3. Autonomic balance. The vegetative nervous system swings between the upshift—in times of stress—and swings back down in times of relaxation.

of organs that are not needed or take away from the response; for this reason, it is called the *Fight or Flight response*. When the sympathetic system is mobilized, it is called *Resistance*. After the stressful stimulus has been managed or has disappeared, sympathetic activation decreases and the parasympathetic reaction increases and is referred to as the *Rest or Digest Response*. During this phase, there may also be an increase in inflammation, as the body aims to *repair* the damage of the previous actions. In other words, the vagal increase is proportional to the activation and length of the resistance phase: The more intense and longer the sympathetic response is, the greater the parasympathetic hypoarousal response.

Depression appears evident during vagal symptom increase and is often accompanied by inflammation (Kop et al., 2010; Schiweck et al., 2019). Before falling into depression, usually there has been a long period of struggling, living in the *resistance* phase, until exhaustion takes over. This is a crucial point: People suffering from depression in most cases are not *weak* or *lazy*, but exhausted because they struggled to continue doing things like before, often refusing to accept inner or outer changes for far too long.

Besides prolonged stress, another dynamic that may lead to depression is avoiding sadness. This seems a paradox because many people suffering from depression are very often sad, but the core point is that *they continue to be sad because they never fully experience sadness* and so they don't manage to *go over the hill* of sad feelings and, in this way, remain in the grip of sadness.

This dynamic has many practical consequences for therapy because the primary aim is not only to solve the depressed mood state but also to restore the sympathetic–parasympathetic rhythm. Antidepressants may be useful when the person is completely out of the window of tolerance and it is not possible to restore the balance with other nonpharmacological interventions. But this is only for the time necessary to activate and consolidate the nonpharmacological interventions. This is a *strategic* use of medication aiming at restoring natural adaptive resources. If antidepressants are used *not to feel*, or to escape emotions, they lead to chronic depression. Too often in clinical practice, we see antidepressant drugs prescribed for lengthy periods of time, without promoting healthy lifestyles or psychotherapy support. In most of the cases, if nothing has changed, the person will relapse in time, maybe convincing themselves that they cannot be without medication. Depressive disorders require very long treatments, when they do not engage in a person-centered comprehensive program (Sarris et al., 2014).

We must also consider that sympathetic and parasympathetic are synergistic and if we just act on one phase without considering the general rhythm, we may increase mood oscillations, as in in the bipolar spectrum. If an antidepressant drug is prescribed to reduce symptoms in an inappropriate way, it may lead to chronic depression or result in mania.

STABILIZATION

BODY SCREENING OF THE POLYVAGAL STATE: THE SELF-CONTACT TECHNIQUE

In this technique (Box 3.1), therapists accompany patients in a guided exploration that allows them to encounter themselves in an accepting way. At the same time, it is a mode of screening their emotional self-regulation and their ability to be grounded and stable in their daily lives. The versatility of this intervention allows it to be carried out both when people are seen for the first time and in situations of urgency; for example, it has been widely used in emergency contexts such as in the emergency department or in interventions on site with earthquake victims. In a short time and without having to have any specific information about the history of the person, staying in contact with themselves allows therapists to understand not what really happened in people's lives but *the result of what people did with what happened and their current condition.* It is not a way to diagnose patients, but an index of their current state and whether we can proceed reprocessing the trauma or if we need to help with their stabilization techniques, before proceeding with the DeprEnd Protocol.

Psychoeducational Text on the Self-Contact Technique

The Self-Contact Technique provides a brief, simple moment with ourselves. We dedicate ourselves to this moment by taking care of ourselves, experiencing the sensations of contact with our hands and following our internal breathing rhythm, with simplicity and tenderness, as we would toward a loved one. There is nothing to achieve, nothing that must happen, just simply listening and accepting what happens with sensitivity and curiosity, even in the moments when we feel discomfort or nothing seems to happen.

The goal is not relaxation, though this often happens, but inner freedom to be how we truly are, moment by moment, because inner calm is a consequence of this freedom. We truly try to experience it just like an intimate encounter with a person we love: Most of the time it will bring us tranquillity, but also difficult moments are part of friendship. Practically everyone is able to accept us when we are in shape, but only true friends are close to us when we are feeling anxious. We will be happier when a loved one feels well, but we will feel even closer when they do not. A real relationship is created by taking small steps, day after day, accepting both pleasure and suffering, the moments in which we feel in contact and those in which we feel more detached, in a supportive atmosphere. Experiencing it deepens esteem and trust, toward the other person and toward ourselves. We can do even just a part of this practice of friendship every time we want to get closer to ourselves. A particularly important moment is the evening when we are in bed with the lights out and we have nothing else to do, in that very intimate moment just before falling asleep. If we fall asleep while listening to our body, it means we fell asleep close to ourselves. When we sleep, we rely on our subconscious: Free from having to carry out activities in our external life, our subconscious can deal with our inner world, processing the emotions and sensations we have experienced. The dream phase is particularly important: We all dream every night whether we remember them or not; our brain is very active during dreams and works for us, to rebuild our inner balance and give us back our resources to live our lives. The more we can trustfully abandon ourselves to our inner part, the more our sleep will be restful; instead, the more difficulty we have letting go of the control, the more our sleep will be disturbed and less restful. Dedicating this moment of intimate contact before sleeping allows us to be in a close relationship with ourselves when we fall asleep, placing a seed of friendship in our dreams that will bear fruit over time.

Chapter 3   Preparation and Stabilization in EMDR Therapy

> **Box 3.1.** Instructions for the Self-Contact Technique

Rest your hands on your belly, one below and one above the navel, openly and with acceptance.

For at least five consecutive breaths, listen to your breath itself and to the sensations that the contact of your hands on your body transmits to you, accepting them as they are, in any form they may be.

Now, bring the hand that was resting above the naval up onto the chest, onto the area that feels best for you, openly and with acceptance. Listen to the breath that flows between the two hands like a wave and to the sensations that this contact transmits over the course of at least five breaths.

Now, place both hands on your chest, one crossed over the other, feeling where the best place to rest your palms is for you: This may be in the center of your chest, in a higher position between your shoulders, or crossed on your arms. Listen to your breath and to the sensations that this contact with your hands transmits for at least five breaths.

If you wish you can ask yourself: *If the sensations transmitted to me by my hands could talk, what would they tell me?* If a message of support emerges, stay with that, while you listen to your breath.

Now you can choose where to place your hands, it may be both on the abdomen, or on the abdomen and the chest, or both on the chest, wherever they feel best for you, openly and with acceptance. Listen to all the phases of your breath, as if it were a flowing wave, and to the sensations that this contact transmits to you for at least five breaths.

If you feel open to doing so, you can try offering thanks to yourself—bearing in mind the commitment you make each day, as much as possible, to live and help live. Saying thank you does not depend on anything you may have done or did not do; it is deeper than that, directed at the person within who has always tried to do whatever you could, using the tools and the possibilities you had at your disposal, and who each day, as much as you can, really tries to live and help live; in essence, this task represents the <u>life mission</u> that is shared by all of mankind!

And now—if you wish—you can say, slowly: *Dear* (then say your own name), *thank you for everything that you are, thank you so much for everything that you are.*

You can repeat it three to four times, slowly and listening to at least one breath in between each time, saying again: *Dear* (then say your own name), *thank you for everything that you are, thank you so much for everything that you are.*

Note whether even just a small part of you feels the authenticity of the gratitude, but without any expectations and accepting whatever happens, as it will be different each time. For some breaths, listen to your breath and to the sensations that your hands transmit to you though their contact on your body; notice whether you sense anything different compared to the beginning of the practice, accepting whatever comes for what it is.

Now, let your hands rest wherever they feel most comfortable, for example, on your lap or on your legs, for at least five breaths, or for as many as you would like, listen to the air that flows in and out of your body, trying to accept yourself simply and amicably, free to be as you are.

See Figure 3.4 for positions of the Self-Contact Technique.

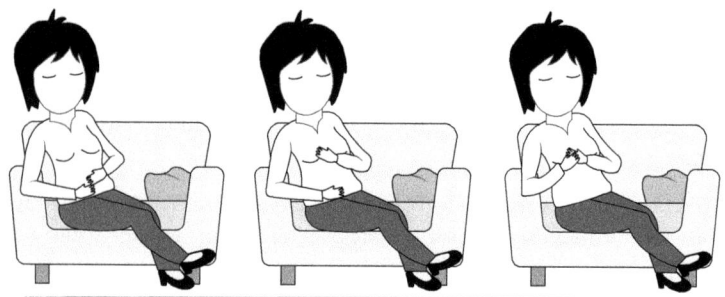

FIGURE 3.4. Positions for the Self-Contact Technique. Notice the different hand positions.

This practice can be seen both as a screening and stabilization technique. It also provides us with an element of verification of possible dissociative disorders. We can use this practice as a *traffic light* that suggests to us how to proceed:

- *Green Light:* When people feel the contact of their feet with the ground and perceive the contact of their hands with their body as protective or warm, we can proceed in the processing of traumas with the protocol because, according to the Polyvagal Theory of Porges, we are in the Affiliation System, capable of containment and empathy and with the knowledge that the five senses are open.
- *Yellow Light:* Initially, people do not feel the contact of their feet with the ground and/or the contact of their hands with the body is uncomfortable. By performing stabilization techniques, such as grounding, alignment, or centering, they are able to re-access the contact of their feet with the ground and comfortable contact of their hands on their body. From the Polyvagal Theory perspective, this indicates activation of the sympathetic Fight–Flight response, but with the ability to re-access the ability to affiliate/connect. In this case, we can proceed with emotional processing but we must make sure to keep the arousal limited and monitor that the person remains within the window of tolerance.

- *Red Light:* if people do not feel the contact of their feet with the ground or the contact of their hands on their body, stabilization practices are implemented. However, if there is no improvement in the connection with oneself or there is deterioration, it indicates that the time is not yet right for emotional processing of traumatic events and we must continue to work on stabilization techniques and self-regulation. From the Polyvagal Theory perspective, it corresponds to the block/submission state and the diagnostic probability of a dissociative disorder, even if the practice itself does not allow the formal diagnosis of it. The red light can also occur in emotional situations in which the person is outside the window of tolerance, and is not necessarily dissociative. Conversely, when there is dissociation, there is almost always a red light, so it is a highly sensitive and helpful technique. It is important to remember that it only indicates the current state, not the structural one.

In addition to being a screening technique, it is also an important stabilization technique, because it can help patients regain their centrality and recover a sense of connection and can also pave the way to other stabilization practices, such as listening to breathing, grounding, centering, and practicing loving-kindness toward oneself. In addition, this practice can also facilitate and integrate the exercise of the Safe Place in the Standard EMDR Protocol (Shapiro, 2000), if it is done as a preparation for visualization. As we have described, a particularly important moment to practice even a small part of the contact with ourselves is when we are in bed just before falling asleep: Dreams are a very important moment in emotional processing and dedicating a brief moment of emotional contact plants the seed of affectivity into our dreams (Rasch & Born, 2013).

THE ROLE OF DIAPHRAGMATIC BREATHING AND OTHER SOMATIC RESOURCES

Important somatic resources, available at all times, are grounding, alignment, centering (as in the Self-Contact Technique) and above all diaphragmatic breathing. Diaphragmatic breathing is especially important during EMDR processing. When breathing is shallow and in the thoracic region, there are more thoughts, more anxiety, and a reduced ability to process (Caldwell & Victoria, 2011); when breathing is diaphragmatic, it is easier to be in the observer role resulting in less anxiety, fewer thoughts, and stronger processing (Hopper et al., 2019). Many times, blockages can be prevented and overcome during EMDR processing by ensuring that the person—at least partially—maintains a diaphragmatic level of breathing.

Breathing can also be a companion, a safety anchor that the person can turn to at any time. In ordinary conditions, we breathe in a three-stroke rhythm, like a waltz: inhalation, exhalation, the pause between when one breath ends and the other begins.

Most people have no pauses because the state of underlying anxiety, in which we tend to live, does not allow it. This really is a pity because when we reach that moment at the bottom of the exhalation where everything is still, there is a moment of profound peace that gives a different rhythm to what we are experiencing and doing. With the pause, the diaphragm descends, breathing becomes deeper and the underlying anxiety—that blurs everything— disperses, allowing us to perceive more clearly. When there is a pause, we also have a greater probability that our evaluation of events is correct, while when it is lacking there is a greater risk that it is distorted by our prejudices or fears.

Paradoxically, from a physiological point of view, slowing down breathing by reducing breaths per minute increases oxygenation, improving energy and mood and reducing body inflammation. The difference in oxygenation is not how much we inhale at rest, we use less than 15% of the oxygen we inhale the difference is how much oxygen our body extracts from blood. This is much greater if breathing slows down (Russo, 2017). No effort is necessary, it is sufficient to exhale calmly, without hurrying to inhale again and allowing ourself the natural pause, if possible, between one breath and another. All animals that live longer, like the elephant or turtle—who can live for 400 years—have few breaths per minute with pauses between each breath! If we breathe shallowly, at chest level, we will take many breaths per minute with reduced oxygenation and increased thoughts and anxiety. If instead, we breathe using the diaphragm, spontaneous breathing slows down, we increase oxygenation, and the spinal column and internal organs are also massaged.

In any case we must not force anything, but only note *if* we can let air be collected by inhaling at the level of the abdomen and sides, instead of in the chest, and allow a small pause between breaths: If this is not possible at the moment, the fact of becoming aware of it and observing it little by little will create the conditions for it to happen spontaneously over time.

DEVELOPING DIAPHRAGMATIC BREATHING

The diaphragm is the main respiratory muscle. When we inhale it moves down, lowering the lobes of the lungs and drawing air inside the abdomen; on exhaling, the lobes of the lungs rise back up and the air is released through this elastic return. When it moves down during inspiration, air fills in the abdomen which expands forward, sideways, and toward the spinal column, like a balloon that swells in all directions. Breathing, at the level of the chest, follows when there is a need for additional energy, such as in physical exertion or when intense emotions are experienced; instead during rest, the air that is drawn by the diaphragmatic movement is largely sufficient, so that the chest is stationary or subsequently expands, in a limited way, as an extension of the diaphragmatic movement (Ogden & Fisher, 2015).

To help us in recognizing this, we can place our hands on our abdomen and our chest, as in the practice of the Self-Contact Technique, noting if the abdomen expands and the chest is stationary or expands later in a lesser way. We also note if we perceive our sides expanding, while the abdomen slightly swells outward; even just a small movement can be enough.

To further improve our awareness of the diaphragm moving, we can sit down and bend forward, leaning our elbows on our legs with our face looking toward the floor a few meters before us. In this position, the chest movement tends to be partially blocked while that of the diaphragm is more evident: Breathing normally we try to become aware that while we inhale, the diaphragm moves down and air collects, the abdomen and sides expand and they release during exhaling. We also note if we can perceive a slight expansion at the level of the lumbar spine, which tends to flatten when air collects and recover its curvature when air is released.

Let's not worry if we do not perceive it; it is enough to perceive even a slight movement, observing what happens without forcing anything: It is an awareness experiment, it is not necessary to change anything that is happening! Now we can go back to the sitting position and note if we can perceive the diaphragm moving, even slightly, through the expansion of the abdomen and sides. If it can help, we can place a hand on one side, under the costal arch for a few breaths to increase movement sensitivity. If it is difficult to perceive the expansion, we can go back to the previous position for a few breaths to regain awareness.

Breathing with the diaphragm initially requires attention, but if we try two to three times a day for a few minutes (3 or 5) every day, it becomes automatic after a few weeks and we will feel the benefits such as the reduction of anxiety, more stabilization and concentration capacity, as well as improving the efficacy of the emotional processing protocol.

Important: Do these experiments with curiosity, exploring what happens without worrying about achieving a result. We experiment with the various positions, opening receptivity to physical sensations without needing to force anything.

Let's remember that the diaphragm works for us anyway, whether we perceive it or not, because this is the mission it received from life. If we can recognize it a little at a time, it will become a trusted friend and we will be able to feel it *with us* every time we regain the awareness of breathing.

In Box 3.2 are two examples of other somatic resources.

Box 3.2. Examples of Somatic Resources: Instructions for Grounding and Alignment Resources

Grounding: Gently become aware of your body. Notice if you can relax your forehead and face; notice if you can relax your shoulders, arms, and hands; notice if you can relax your trunk; now notice if you can relax your legs and feet. Note your posture and feel the contact between you and the ground. Feel the support of the firm surface where you are. Be conscious of your feet and toes—their shape, consistency—note what points of the feet are in contact with the ground and which have been released—breathe out and let yourself go into the ground, and each time you breathe out, let yourself go even more deeply into the ground—push down gently and plant the right foot into the ground—feel the resistance of the firm surface that supports them—the muscles contracting during the light pressure—then let go—feeling the relaxation—now push down gently and plant the left foot into the ground—feel the resistance of the ground—the muscles contracting during the light pressure—then let go—you can alternate pressure, contraction, then release with one foot—then with the other one—then you can notice the quality of the contact of both feet on the ground, and each time you breathe out, let yourself go even more deeply in the ground.

Alignment: Gently become aware of your body. Note your posture and feel the contact between you and the ground. Be conscious of your feet and how they support your ankles. Your ankles that support your legs. Your legs that support your pelvis. Be aware of your pelvis that supports your lower back—your lower back that supports your upper back—your upper back that supports your neck and head. Try gently to rotate the pelvis forward, noticing how your back stretches—imagine that there's a thread that is pulling you up from the neck and head, pulling them up—each time air flows out, your shoulders fall toward the ground—your neck and head extend slightly upward—a little more each time that air flows out. With the next breath out, relax your shoulders and extend your back toward the sky, in a position that inspires dignity—be aware of being right here—right now.

GLIMPSING THE "HIDDEN HEART:" THE "MAGIC QUERY"

The most painful aspect of depression is often the loss of the ability to love, which is particularly painful when it concerns loved ones like children or family members (Risch et al., 2009; Yap et al., 2014). In these cases, people can attack themselves for this lack of feeling and this contributes to worsening the depression. The situation can be so difficult that sometimes people need something magical in order to hope to transform it. In the following practice we try to help them find something magical in themselves.

It is a simple but useful practice both as a diagnostic assessment and as psychoeducation to help a person who is going through a depressive moment to see the light at the end of the tunnel. Ask this question:

If by magic you could freely choose what you would like to feel toward yourself, what would you really like to feel?

It is important to underline that we are asking the person to think about not what they feel now toward themselves, but, if they were really free to choose, using a magic wand, what they would like to feel toward themselves. We ask them not to answer straight away but to try to listen to their inner self, while we do bilateral brief tapping on the hands or with eye movements. If we are not yet certain that a person is ready to receive tapping, we can let them listen to the answer to this question with their eyes closed. Most people answer that they would like to feel self-esteem, friendship, or affection toward themselves. In this case the patient is asked to focus on this and use one or two brief sets of tapping sets.

Note: Some patients find it hard to think about themselves positively, so if addressed to patients with this issue, ask them to do this *without suffering any damage*, because often they are afraid of getting hurt if they allow themselves to feel positive feelings.

After having installed the feelings that they would like to feel, a metaphor is proposed, asking patients to listen to it (preferably with their eyes closed), accompanied by light tapping.

In winter, if you look at a lawn from the outside everything looks dry and barren, there are only a few dry plants. This can be similar to depressive periods where everything seems to have lost its vitality. However, in that winter soil, below the ground there are the seeds of plants and flowers that remain hidden and protected pending the arrival of spring. This is similar to the hearts of the people who are facing the winter of depression and are hidden behind a protective shell to protect the most delicate part of themselves. From the outside, apparently everything seems gray and barren, but inside the heart is alive and is waiting for the return of the new spring in which feelings and colors will return. Through this little magical question, you can learn to look into your heart that may be hidden in the shell of winter of depression, waiting to reopen when conditions will allow.

The answer to what we would like to feel is much truer than the absence of feelings! If we recognize it, we will have a little more confidence to wait for the return of spring.

A minority of those affected by severe depression do not want to have positive feelings toward themselves because they feel existential guilt, or they have non-integrated self-attack parts as in some dissociative or psychotic disorders (Gambin and Sharp, 2018;

Chapter 3 Preparation and Stabilization in EMDR Therapy

McCanlies et al., 2017). In this case, the answer is diagnostic and suggestive of a deeper psychopathological disorder.

INSTALLING MEMORIES OF RESOURCES FROM THE PAST

When a resource is needed and is missing in the present, we can look if the person experienced it in the past, even only once, and can recover and access these positive feelings in the present.

Even when depressed, often we have *hidden seeds* of resources, waiting silently for the conditions to grow: We have to look more for seeds than for full resources. As a therapist, we can pay attention to whether we feel connected to the person. It doesn't matter if we are not able to label a specific resource, the resource is latent in the relational field and is likely to appear over time.

When we find a seed, we can explore and integrate it, creating a little *secret* connection. One way to do this is—if we feel comfortable—with eye contact with clients allowing them to feel support from the experience. It is useful to install the eye connection resource; it supports the activation of the *Affiliation State* (Porges, 2007; Porges & Furman, 2011).

Case Study 3.1

USING HAKOMI'S 3-STEP PROCEDURE WITH A DEPRESSED ADULT FEMALE

Lidia is a 58-year-old social worker, married, with one son living in another country with his wife. She was born in a region of Italy with a traditional culture. At the beginning of the therapy, she had been suffering from depression for about 5 years, with some improvement with antidepressant therapy but without recovering the pleasure of life. When recounting her history, she said that, even if depression came later, she started to lose pleasure soon after her wedding. She was the last of a large family and she never felt nurtured by her mother; her father was her affective support. She had an affectionate relationship with her husband, but in spite of that she continued to feel worthless.

In the following session, I asked her to let the words *I'm worth it* resonate inside and float back slowly in the past, listening to her breathing, noticing if she experienced that, even if only once during her past.

From a technical point of view, I often use the *3-Step Procedure* derived from the Hakomi Method (Kurtz, 1990) and Sensorimotor Psychotherapy (Ogden & Fisher, 2015) by alternating the following:

- *Contact Statement (CS):* Use a statement to contact to the present moment experience, mirroring what the person says or shows nonverbally.

- *Mindfulness Directive (MD):* "Stay with that ..." with bilateral stimulation (BLS).
- *Mindfulness Exploration (ME):* Do ME by asking a question without a direct answer, listening to what comes up inside during BLS.

This is a very powerful way to slow the pace and help to develop mindful dual consciousness of the present moment experience, increasing connection and expanding the window of tolerance with the past target. The BLS increases the rhythm and the efficacy of the process.

P (Patient): My Dad's memory comes to mind, beside the relationship I had with my Daddy, I was the youngest of his daughters, he called me his little child, then I remember he cuddled me, he put me on his knees and he told me stories of when he was at war and things like that.	
T (Therapist): Do you feel like staying with this?	
P: (She nods). It is nice, because I remember, I don't know how to explain, I was feeling as if I were more important than the others, because he was holding me on his knees, we were near the fireplace in the countryside.	
T: More important than the others.	CS
P: And he used to tell me (tales), because my brothers and sisters were also there on their chairs, but I was the youngest and he used to hold me in his arms.	
T: How old are you in this image that is coming up now?	
P: 6 to 7 years old.	
T: How about if we stay with that?	
P: It is something joyful, happy.	

T: Well, this little child feels that joy, that happiness. Stay with that joy, this happiness. BLS	CS MD. Slow the pace and gradually activate the present moment experience.
P: A joy as … you know, when someone says to the others: "Look, he's holding me in his arms and not you."	
T: Well, he holds her in his arms and not the others. Stay with the little child's sensation while her father is holding her in his arms and not the others. BLS	CS (continue stimulation) MD
T: What does this little child learn about herself from the fact that he holds her in his arms and not the others? BLS	ME. Exploring the resource gently, without a direct answer but asking to feel inside.
P: Protection.	Positive Cognition (PC)
T: Protection. BLS	CS
T: If this protection could speak, what would it say to the child about herself? BLS	ME: Deepening the experience.
P: I'm important for my daddy.	
T: I'm important for my Daddy. Stay with this belief that arises in the little child while her father holds her in his arms: *I'm important.* BLS How is it for the little child to let this belief, learned from her father, of *I'm important* resonate inside? BLS	CS MD
P: Happiness.	
T: Stay with that happiness. BLS	

Now we will try to do something. Say goodbye to the little child, telling her that we will come back to her, and then let this belief, that she learned from her father, of *I'm important* resonate inside. See if there is even a single little moment in your present life when you feel it again, even only little moments when you feel *I'm important* comes back.
BLS

| | Float forward in mindful state, exploring the seed of the resource in present life. |

P: My little niece.

T: Your little niece.
Stay with the image that comes of your little niece when you feel you are important.

CS
MD

BLS

P: My little niece embraces me, and she says to me that she needs me, and she loves me.

T: Very well; your little niece embraces you and says to you that she loves you.
Stay with that, when your little niece embraces you and says to you that she loves you.
BLS

CS
MD

P: It seems that my heart should burst, I don't know how to explain it.
(I feel) Tranquillity, my little child is embracing me.

T: Tranquillity, the little child embracing you, the belief that you learned a long time ago of *I'm important* resonating inside you.
Stay with that.
BLS

CS
MD

Which emotions come while you see your little niece embracing you and you feel *I'm important* resonate inside?
BLS

Chapter 3 Preparation and Stabilization in EMDR Therapy

P: I also feel a bit of fear.

T: Yes. Is there only fear or is there something else too?

P: I'm afraid one day this might end.

T: Sure, there is fear, and we'll deal with it, but is there only fear now or is there some pleasant emotion, too?
BLS

P: No, there is also joy because I feel important and happy to see that my little niece loves me.

T: Certainly, we'll take care of your fear, but now can we stay exclusively with that part of joy, only with that today? | We're working on the resource; we briefly contact fear but make an agreement that we will deal with it later and go back to the resource.

P: Yes.

T: Stay with that joy while you let the belief, *I'm important*, resonate inside.
BLS | MD

P: The strength.

T: The strength.

P: The strength that my niece gives me. | CS

T: Very well, feel the strength that your niece gives you.
BLS | MD

If this strength, which goes along with the belief *I'm important*, could express itself through a gesture or a movement, what kind of movement or gesture would it be?
BLS

| Expanding the experience of the resource: from feeling and cognition to the body with movement. That latent presence of fear makes movement more protective than feeling body sensations.

P: To embrace my niece.

| The resource is expressing with its energy!

T: Very well. Can you try to do this movement now? Very well. Feel this movement, its sensations, let *I'm important* resonate inside: There is such a rich seed inside you that resurfaces in the encounter with your niece.

| MD deepening of the experience of the resource.

If this movement of embracing, which goes along with this strength and the feeling of *I'm important*, could express itself through a very little movement, a kind of secret movement, that only you know you're doing, while those around you don't notice it, what kind of little movement could it be, recalling the whole embrace, and known only to you?

| Creating the "Secret Movement" to link to the resource.

P: I don't know.

T: Try to release the embrace by keeping its sensations, going back to the position before the embracing, and now try to do a little movement, that only you know, but that holds the whole embracing, a kind of *secret* movement that belongs only to you.

P: Closing my hand.

| The "secret" movement

T: Does it correspond?

P: (She nods.)

T: Very well.

T: Now can you open your hand and then slowly close it as you let the words *I'm important* resonate inside? What do you notice, as you do it?	Integrating gesture and PC.
P: I feel more … as if I had strength, the strength to react.	
T: Very well. Stay with that strength of reacting while you feel your hand closing and let the words *I'm important* resonate inside. BLS OK. Do you feel like doing it once more?	MD
P: (She nods.)	
T: Open your hand and close it while you recall the sensations of the embracing and let *I'm important* resonate, as a vibration in the body that resonates while your hand is closing, let *I'm important* resonate sometimes while you feel your hand closing. What do you notice now?	Deepening the resource
P: Courage.	
T: Very well. Stay with this courage. Now imagine being in your daily life and you do it without anyone realizing it. BLS	MD Connecting to everyday life keeping it as a "secret" resource.
What do you notice as you imagine doing it in your daily life?	
P: A sense of strength and courage.	
T: Well, stay with this sense of strength and courage. BLS I would try something more. Can you open your eyes, open your hand, and do it again while you look at me? Do you feel we are connected?	MD Exploring the experience of installing the resource with eye connection. Verifying connection before doing the gesture.

P: Yes.	
T: Very well. Can you do it again? That is, slowly close your hand as you let the words *I'm important* resonate inside? I'll close my hand, too, while you do it, and inside me, as we look at each other, I'll let the words *I'm important* resonate so we'll hold it together. OK? Give me the start. Very well. What is it like doing it together?	Installation, mirroring the client's resource.
P: (She nods with pleasure.)	
T: Perfect. One last time, can you still do it? One last time, we'll do it together and I'll support that seed inside you. Very well. What is the sensation like?	Once again
P: Beautiful.	
T: As you have just seen, you can also do it when you look at people with your eyes open, whenever you want, you don't need to close your eyes, and this allows you to use it any time you want.	
P: And it gives strength.	
T: Nobody realizes it, only you know it, and you have a seed inside that, when nourished, can really grow, a seed that was sowed a long time ago.	
P: With my Dad.	
T: With your Dad.	
P: And I'm not worthless anymore, if my father loved me so, and my niece shows me so much, it means that I'm worth it, I'm not useless!	
At the next session:	
T: Did you use your movement?	

> **P:** Yes, and it works well enough, yes. Because it feels like I detach from everything and I say, *I'm important.*
>
> **T:** When did you use it?
>
> **P:** During a discussion with my husband concerning usual matters, other times when I was suffering, and then with my son.
>
> **T:** Very well. Can you use it once a day, every day? Even if there is nothing that makes it necessary?
>
> **P:** I didn't think of that.
>
> **T:** Just like a seed to cultivate and so, as a little plant that needs some water every day, by recalling it every day you help it to grow.
>
> **P:** Yes.

REGULATING THE AROUSAL: THE LEAVE AND RECALL TECHNIQUE

It is a simple and very effective practice to regulate arousal during EMDR processing. It derives from the *Two Tugs* technique by Knipe, causing the person to oscillate between the contact with the traumatic material and the recovery of a state of security, but is carried out more quickly during bilateral stimulation (BLS).

The principle is this: When the patient goes outside their window of tolerance during BLS, they are asked to let go of the image and, while continuing the BLS, remain focused only on the movement of the therapist's fingers, the discomfort in their body, and their breathing. By doing this, there is normally a recovery of their stability. After the set, they are asked what they notice and then using the image of the target, reprocessing can be resumed. If the person stays within the window of tolerance, we proceed according to the classic protocol, otherwise we repeat the *leave and recall technique*.

Leaving the Remote Control to Patients

After letting patients experience leaving the image, focusing only on the eye movements and on breathing a couple of times, there is a rapid recovery of a state of stability, and the therapist can leave the operation of the remote control to patients:

> *Have you noticed that when you leave the image and follow only the fingers, your activation/discomfort decreases rapidly? So far, I have chosen how long you stay in contact*

with the image, now I will let you do it. Stay in contact for as long as you can tolerate it because it helps to process the event more thoroughly. When you feel the activation is increasing to a level you feel you cannot tolerate, leave the image, continuing to just follow the fingers, and as you have experienced, and the activation will decrease.

If patients decide to leave the image, they must not recall the image in that set, but in the following one. Most frequently, what happens when they start using the *remote control* the first time is that patients leave the image to check that the discomfort is really reduced—similar to when therapists ask clients to stop, take a breath, after a set is completed. Once they have checked that there is a decrease in their discomfort and it reduces when they do it, it is interesting that, afterward, nearly no one ends up leaving the image and they stay in contact with it for the entire duration of the BLS. This greatly increases the person's resilience and their ability to stay in contact with emotions!

During the protocol, patients are in the hands of their therapists and even if they are given the stop signal to warn us if they are in too much discomfort, they are afraid that they will have to suffer too much. Through the leave and recall technique, patients experience that, if the discomfort becomes too much, they can quickly regain control and this generates more of a sense of self-efficacy and strength.

Furthermore, there is a positive effect on relationships. In EMDR, one of the major risks—at the transference level—is that therapists are experienced in an idealized way and this could accentuate pre-existing attachment problems: If patients have a dependent disorder, they tend to become even more dependent on their therapists; if instead they have an avoidant tendency, their fear of being under the control of their therapists can increase. Making patients more autonomous within an empathic relationship reduces the transferential distortion and increases the therapeutic alliance on a healthier and more collaborative level.

In applying the *leave and recall technique*, different levels of protection can be used that allow for reducing contact with the traumatic material. This depends on if there is necessity to recover the window of tolerance. Over time, it supports the return to the Standard EMDR Protocol (Shapiro, 2018). There are three levels of protection:

- *Level 1 Protection:* We keep the focus on the image and the bodily location of the discomfort for a short time, then we leave the image and continue only with eye movements, body location, and breathing. In subsequent sets, the contact time is progressively increased, until the image can be kept for the whole time.
- *Level 2 Protection:* If the arousal is higher or the tolerance is reduced, the image is not recalled, but focus remains only on the eye movements and breathing.
- *Level 3 Protection:* In the case of an even higher arousal or very low tolerance, focus is only on eye movements with neither bodily location nor breathing.

When people tolerate affect to a greater extent, they go back to the Standard EMDR Protocol, where they are in contact with the image, with the negative cognition and body location.

An interesting aspect is that the eye movements act as stabilizers regarding both hyperarousal and hypoarousal; therefore, the leave and recall technique can be used in both states. Maintaining awareness of diaphragmatic breathing during the processing, even if only in part, increases emotional containment, as well as the awareness of contact with the ground and the chair and a relatively aligned posture.

Case Study 3.2

USING THE LEAVE AND RECALL TECHNIQUE

The client is the mother of a 16-year-old girl who was abused during a holiday at the sea side. The session focuses on the worst episode, when she discovered what happened to her daughter.
Note: BLS, bilateral stimulation; CS, contact statement; MD, mindfulness directive; ME, mindfulness exploration; NC, negative cognition; PC, positive cognition.

P (Patient): The sensation I felt when I was doing yoga on the shore. I turned around and I saw my daughter who had just had a shower and she had moved closer to her daddy and she was crying. I was afraid that something had happened to her.	
T (Therapist): So, the moment when you saw her crying after her shower is something that causes you pain while you think of it.	CS
P: Yes.	
T: Take a deep breath.	
P: She was asking me: *Mum, why was he hurting me, and asking me if I liked it?*	
T: And this is, as you think of it, what hurts you most?	CS
Do you feel that we can work on that?	Asking for permission
P: I never answered her.	
T: You never answered her.	CS
(Assessment of Negative Cognition [NC], Positive Cognition [PC])	
Which emotion are you feeling now?	
P: Pain.	

T: Pain.
And while you look at this image and let the words *I'm not able to protect* resonate and you feel this pain, how strong is the discomfort now? On a scale of 0 to 10, where 0 is no disturbance or neutral and 10 is the highest disturbance you can imagine, how disturbing does the memory feel to you now?

P: 10.

T: Where do you feel it in your body?

P: (Indicates chest.)

T: You feel it in your chest. Please look at my fingers, recall the image and the words *I'm not able to protect*, and feel this pain in your chest. OK? Now leave the image, follow only my fingers, while listening to your breathing … only the fingers and the breathing.	Emotional pain increases until the edge of the window of tolerance: LEAVE AND RECALL TECHNIQUE Level 2 Protection
P: I feel pain. T: You feel much pain in your chest. Look at my fingers, listen only to the breathing while you follow my fingers without the image … now only the fingers and the breathing.	CS LEAVE AND RECALL TECHNIQUE Level 2 Protection
P: I'm breathing.	
T: Very well. Recall the image as it appears now. What do you notice in your body? BLS Now leave the image and follow only my fingers. Only my fingers.	LEAVE AND RECALL TECHNIQUE Level 3 Protection
P: I feel better.	
T: Take a deep breath. Did you notice if there is any difference when you notice the image and when I tell you to leave it and follow only my fingers?	

P: Yes.

T: What does it change?

P: That it makes me relax.

T: When you leave the image?

P: Yes.

T: Very well. Until now, I have decided how long to stay in contact with the image and when to leave it and follow only my fingers. Now I will leave the remote controller with you. The more you notice the image, the more we process what has occurred so, as far as you can tolerate it and it is not too strong, keep the image as it is; when you feel it is getting too strong leave the image and follow only my fingers. Now I will leave you the control of how long to notice the image and when to leave it.
BLS | LEAVING THE REMOTE CONTROLLER

P: ...

T: What do you notice with the image?

P: That I was afraid for her.

T: OK. Let's try to go back to the episode we started with.
BLS
What do you notice now?

P: Pain.

T: There is pain in your body as you recall it now. Where do you feel it? | CS

P: In my chest.

T: Let's stay with that, OK? Remember, as much as you feel you can, stay in contact with the image. When you feel the suffering is getting too strong, leave it and follow only my fingers.
BLS
What do you notice now?

| | Leaving the remote controller |

P: I had to detach myself from the memory because it was hurting me here, but now I feel better.

| | She experimented that detaching from the image the suffering decreased. |

T: Very well.
How do you notice that you are feeling better now?

P: I can breathe better.

T: OK.
BLS

P: I feel anger.

T: You feel anger.
Stay with that.
BLS

| | CS |

P: I'm very angry now.

T: OK. Stay with your anger.
BLS.

P: That I feel more and more anger.

T: Stay with your anger.
BLS

P: There is sadness.

T: Sadness.
Stay with this sadness.
BLS
Where do you feel this sadness in your body?

| | CS |

Chapter 3 Preparation and Stabilization in EMDR Therapy

P: In the chest.	
T: Can you stay in contact with this sadness, feel it in the chest? While breathing through it? Do you feel like resting your hands on your knees? Letting your arms relax? BLS	MD
Stay in contact with your sadness in your chest while you listen to your breathing. BLS	
Leave the image. Listen only to the alternate tapping and breathing. BLS What do you notice now?	LEAVE AND RECALL TECHNIQUE Level 2 Protection
P: That I'm tired. T: You are very tired, of course. Can you look at my fingers only, without recalling the episode? Only my fingers. BLS	LEAVE AND RECALL TECHNIQUE Level 3 Protection to recover from hypoarousal
P: I'm getting relaxed.	
T: Very well, go with that. BLS	
P: (She seems surprised.)	
T: What did you notice when you tried to recall the episode?	
P: That I can't remember.	
T: That you can't remember. Go with that.	
P: I feel relaxed.	
T: Ok. Good.	

EMDR AND LIFESTYLES: WALKING WITH TWO LEGS

Lifestyle changes are an essential component of an integrated approach to treatment for depression. Research on major depression has confirmed that it's caused by an array of biopsychosocial and lifestyle factors. Diet, physical activity, and sleep play a significant mediating role in the development, progression, and treatment of depression (Berk et al., 2013; Lopresti et al., 2013; Sarris et al., 2014). A recent study highlighted that supporting lifestyle changes for sleep hygiene, physical activity, diet, and sunlight exposure improves the outcomes of standard antidepressant treatment (Garcia-Toro et al., 2012). A heuristic, theoretical framework explains how the modern lifestyle may impact mental health. Obesity (Luppino et al., 2010), poor diet (Jacka et al., 2010), poor/decreased sleep (Roth, 2004), exposure to chemicals and pollutants (Lim et al., 2012), and high-stress levels (Van Praag, 2004) may potentially disrupt the hypothalamic–pituitary–adrenal (HPA) axis, increase cortisol, and increase low-grade systemic inflammation and oxidative stress. Both neuroendocrine disruption and inflammation have been linked to the etiology of depression (Maes et al., 2012; Raison et al., 2006).

Physical Activity

Depression is commonly associated with low levels of physical activity. Epidemiological studies have shown that adequate physical activity (PA), based on clinical guidelines, is associated with fewer depressive symptoms, while insufficient PA may be a risk factor for the development of depressive symptoms (Sarris et al., 2014). Moreover, several reviews and meta-analyses showed the efficacy of exercise as a treatment for depression (Knapen et al., 2015; Lopresti et al., 2013). Physical activity interventions had a moderate inhibitory effect on depressive symptoms in adults with and without clinical depression (Conn, 2010), also compared with antidepressant medications (Carek et al., 2011) and with cognitive behavioral therapy (Rimer et al., 2012). In particular, for mild to moderate depression, the effect of exercise may be comparable to antidepressant medication and psychotherapy, while for severe depression exercise seems to be a valuable complementary therapy to the traditional treatments (Knapen et al., 2015). Exercise provides beneficial effects to the neuroendocrine systems (e.g., by stimulating the body to produce serotonin and endorphins; Moylan et al., 2013), and it also increases self-efficacy and self-esteem, which are important psychological issues among people who are depressed (Deslandes et al., 2009). Furthermore, physical activity may have additional beneficial effects by increasing engagement in social interactions and enhancing body image perceptions.

Diet

Over recent years, evidence has emerged to suggest that poor diet may be a risk factor for the onset of depression. Cross-sectional and prospective studies showed that poor dietary patterns and quality are associated with depressed mood and anxiety (Jacka et al., 2012; Sarris et al., 2014). Adherence to a Mediterranean diet comprising high levels of vegetables, fruit, nuts, cereal, legumes, and fish; a moderate alcohol intake; and a low consumption of meat or meat products and whole-fat dairy are protective factors against the development of depression (Sánchez-Villegas et al., 2009). A recent meta-analysis (Li et al., 2017) evaluated the relationship between dietary patterns and the risk of depression, showing that a healthy eating pattern may decrease the risk of depression, whereas Western-style eating patterns may increase the risk of depression. In particular, a healthy dietary pattern, characterized by a high intake of fruit, vegetables, whole grain, fish, olive oil, low-fat dairy, and antioxidants and low intakes of animal foods, was associated with a decreased risk of depression. On the contrary, a Western-style dietary pattern characterized by high consumption of red and/or processed meat, refined grains, sweets, high-fat dairy products, butter, potatoes, and high-fat gravy and low intakes of fruits and vegetables is associated with an increased risk of depression. Various pathways have been proposed that can explain the mechanisms underpinning the association between diet and mental health. Diet modulates several key biological processes that underscore mood disorders, including brain plasticity and function, the stress response system, mitochondria, inflammation, and oxidative processes (Berk & Jacka, 2012). There is now strong evidence in human studies that adherence to a Mediterranean diet is associated with reduced inflammatory markers (Lopresti et al., 2013). Moreover, new intervention studies implementing dietary changes suggest promise for the prevention and treatment of depression (Jacka, 2017). Preliminary evidence now suggests that dietary improvement can both prevent and treat depression (Jacka, 2017; Sarris et al., 2015).

Sleep

In major depression, almost 90% of patients report sleep disturbances (Motivala et al., 2006, Riemann & Voderholzer, 2003). The relationship between insomnia and depression is bidirectional; that is, insomnia can increase depression risk and vice versa (Alvaro et al., 2013). Sleep difficulties increase inflammatory mediators; conversely, elevated inflammatory molecules heighten the risk of sleep problems (Lopresti et al., 2013). Insomnia is also associated with a significantly increased risk of developing a new depressive episode (Baglioni et al., 2011; Taylor et al., 2005), with poorer response to treatment (Dombrovski et al., 2008). Moreover, different studies documented improvements in mood and depressive symptoms following insomnia-specific interventions such as cognitive behavioral therapy for insomnia and mindfulness-based cognitive therapy (Manber et al., 2008). EMDR has also been found to improve sleep in posttraumatic stress disorder (PTSD) sufferers (Raboni et al., 2006, 2014). Additionally, the use of lifestyle modification programs may improve sleep by addressing factors associated with poor sleep; for example, sedentary lifestyle, poor diet, and caffeine and alcohol use (Sarris et al., 2014).

THE SYNERGY OF EMDR AND LIFESTYLE INTERVENTIONS IN DEPRESSION

Studies showed that providing only written recommendations on lifestyle is not sufficient for depressed patients to benefit from it, so it is important to consider how to present the lifestyle modification recommendations to patients and the importance of monitoring systems for their implementation (Serrano Ripoll et al., 2015). It is essential, in the initial evaluation, to analyze physical activity, breathing, diet, sleep, and sociability. It is important to educate concerning these areas and which useful points can be modified and which can have a direct effect on the path of depression. After identifying them, it is helpful to discuss and rank these activities on a scale of up to 10 steps from the easiest to modify to the most difficult. The order is not primarily based on the importance of the objective but on its feasibility. A gradual approach with depressive patients is much more likely to succeed over time than to attempt multiple steps all at once due to low or absent motivation. Sometimes, at the beginning, it is prudent to not even take any step, but wait for the motivation to grow during the treatment. Also, when patients reach the first step, it is important that they stabilize themselves on that level, before proceeding to the next step. A path that proceeds gradually, by stabilizing one goal at a time, is more effective than facing many goals at one time.

An important phenomenon in EMDR therapy is the fact that, in the period following the processing of a traumatic event, a window opens with a variable duration, generally of 15 to 20 days, in which patients develop a greater motivation to take care of themselves. It is very important to use this *window* to see if it is possible to work with one of the steps concerning self-care before immediately processing another trauma. In this way, alternating the processing of life events with the step-by-step ascent on the *lifestyle scale*, patients are *walking with two legs*. Emotional processing and lifestyle will play a synergistic role integrating physical and emotional improvement. The more you are *walking with two legs*, alternating psychotherapeutic processing with lifestyle activities, the more the path of treatment of depression becomes effective and stable. The greatest risk of depression is represented by relapses; however, being able to integrate lifestyle activities into daily living is one of the strongest ways to prevent patients' relapsing into depression.

It is important that the work on lifestyle is not done in a prescriptive way from the outside, but that it is done interactively with patients respecting the reduced motivation that for a certain period characterizes the emotional state of people with depression. It is important to work on motivation, but also to know how to wait, so that resources and the appropriate attitude are crafted through psychotherapeutic work.

THE END OF THE SESSION: THE TRIPLE THANKSGIVING

The conclusion of a session is important in the process of psychotherapeutic practice. If there remains some time, it is helpful to carry out a stabilization exercise, continuing the dialectic process of stepping into the trauma/adverse experience of the *there and then* and then stepping out of that state to go back into the safety of the *here and now*. Patients learn that they can leave the suffering they experienced during the processing inside the session, without dragging it into their everyday life. In this way, they increase their confidence in being able to encounter, experience, and manage emotions in the session. Furthermore, dedicating the last minutes of the session to stabilization also supports generalizing the learned self-administered practices to become part of their ongoing self-care throughout the time between sessions. Different techniques—such as breathing, imaginative work, visualization, and so forth—can be used based on awareness and depending on the therapist's skill and patient's attitude.

Alongside the *external* practice, chosen among the many possible, we like to combine a moment dedicated to the *internal*, silent practice of *Triple Thanksgiving* for us, as therapists. Gratitude is very important from a human, spiritual, and physiological point of view (Fox et al., 2015; Petrocchi & Couyoumdjian, 2016; Watkins et al., 2009; Yoshimura & Berzins, 2017). According to the studies of Health Rate Variability, the feeling of *gratitude* seems to be the one that leads to *cardiac coherence* (Edwards, 2015; McCraty & Childre, 2004), an optimal autonomic balance index between sympathetic and parasympathetic activation. In the moment of the *Gratitude Experience*, a strong relational connection is made and there is no anxiety or depression. It helps to be able to separate because it provides an emotional value to what we have experienced. Indeed, the feeling of gratitude has a fundamental value in spiritual experience and represents an important clinical resource.

These are the three *Thanksgivings*:

- *First Thanksgiving:* The first Thanksgiving—that we silently formulate within—is addressed to patients for the courage they have had to come to the session to open up emotionally, regardless of how much we think they have been involved or not: They still came and did what they were able to do.

  Thank you for the courage you had to come to the session and to open up emotionally, regardless of what you did; you came and did what you were able to do.

- *Second Thanksgiving:* The second Thanksgiving is aimed at ourselves as therapists, because regardless of whether the session was satisfactory or not, we tried to do the best possible for us by letting us be touched by the patient's emotions in the most open way and to dedicate to them all our competence and resources. It may seem unusual to thank ourselves, especially after a session that we may feel we have not managed properly, but it is important: We turn to a deeper level of what did or didn't happen, to our professional and human commitment, regardless of the results.

  Thanks to me because I did the best I could and was touched by my patient and what (choose correct pronoun) was able to accomplish today. I dedicated to (choose correct pronoun) all of my competence and resources and I am thankful for doing what I could do.

- *Third Thanksgiving:* The third Thanksgiving goes to nature and to life itself that gave us the mission of living and helping others to live, giving us powerful resources such as emotions and relationships to support this purpose. It is surprising how strong the power of relationship and emotions can be; unfortunately, when the protective emotions appear, which, as we have said, are initially uncomfortable, the tendency is to remove them. If we meet them, within the window of tolerance, in a climate of friendship toward ourselves, they actually transform themselves and bring us precisely the resources we need at that moment, toward a state of creative peace and open us to life, others, and ourselves. The third Thanksgiving is precisely aimed at nature, life, and its gifts, as the sign of our belonging to humanity, all with the same needs and desires.

  Thanks to nature and life itself that gave us this mission of living and helping others, giving us powerful resources such as emotions and relationships to support this purpose. These gifts of life and connection with life around us result in a sense of human belonging that connects us with our patients, our colleagues, and the world around us.

REFERENCES

Alvares, G. A., Quintana, D. S., Hickie, I. B., & Guastella, A. J. (2016, March). Autonomic nervous system dysfunction in psychiatric disorders and the impact of psychotropic medications: A systematic review and meta-analysis. *Neuroscience, 41*(2), 89–104. https://doi.org/10.1503/jpn.140217

Alvaro, P. K., Roberts, R. M., & Harris, J. K. (2013). A systematic review assessing bidirectionality between sleep disturbances, anxiety, and depression. *Sleep, 36*(7), 1059–1068. https://doi.org/10.5665/sleep.2810

Baglioni, C., Battagliese, G., Feige, B., Spiegelhalder, K., Nissen, C., Voderholzer, U., Lombardo, C., & Riemann, D. (2011). Insomnia as a predictor of depression: A meta-analytic evaluation of longitudinal epidemiological studies. *Journal of Affective Disorders, 135*(1), 10–19. https://doi.org/10.1016/j.jad.2011.01.011

Berk, M., & Jacka, F. (2012). Preventive strategies in depression: Gathering evidence for risk factors and potential interventions. *British Journal of Psychiatry, 201*, 339–341. https://doi.org/10.1192/bjp.bp.111.107797

Berk, M., Sarris, J., Coulson, C. E., & Jacka, F. N. (2013). Lifestyle management of unipolar depression. *Acta Psychiatrica Scandinavica, 2013*(443), 38–54. https://doi.org/10.1111/acps.12124

Berthoz, S., Ouhayoun, B., Parage, N., Kirzenbaum, M., Bourgey, M., & Allilaire, J. (2000). Preliminary study of the levels of emotional awareness in depressed patients and controls. *Annales Medico-Psychologiques, 158*, 665–672. https://doi.org/10.3758/BRM.42.2.586

Boals, A. (2018). Trauma in the eye of the beholder: Objective and subjective definitions of trauma. *Journal of Psychotherapy Integration, 28*(1), 77. https://doi.org/10.1037/int0000050

Braunstein, L. M., Gross, J. J., & Ochsner, K. N. (2017). Explicit and implicit emotion regulation: A multi-level framework. *Social Cognitive and Affective Neuroscience, 12*(10), 1545–1557. https://doi.org/10.1093/scan/nsx096

Caldwell, C., & Victoria, H. K. (2011). Breathwork in body psychotherapy: Toward a more unified theory and practice. *Body Movement and Dance Psychotherapy, 6*(2), 89–101. https://doi.org/10.1080/17432979.2011.574505

Carek, P. J., Laibstain, S. E., & Carek, S. M. (2011). Exercise for the treatment of depression and anxiety. *International Journal of Psychiatry in Medicine, 41*, 15–28. https://doi.org/10.2190/PM.41.1.c

Conn, V. S. (2010). Depressive symptom outcomes of physical activity interventions: Meta-analysis findings. *Annals of Behavioral Medicine, 39*(2), 128–138. https://doi.org/10.1007/s12160-010-9172-x

Corrigan, F. M., Fisher, J. J., & Nutt, D. J. (2011). Autonomic dysregulation and the window of tolerance model of the effects of complex emotional trauma. *Journal of Psychopharmacology, 25*(1), 17–25. https://doi.org/10.1177/0269881109354930

Deslandes, A., Moraes, H., Ferreira, C., Veiga, H., Silveira, H., Mouta, R., Pompeu, F. A., Coutinho, E. S., & Laks, J. (2009). Exercise and mental health: Many reasons to move. *Neuropsychobiology, 59*(4), 191–198. https://doi.org/10.1159/000223730

Dombrovski, A. Y., Cyranowski, J. M., Mulsant, B. H., Houck, P. R., Buysse, D. J., Andreescu, C., Thase, M. E., Mallinger, A. G., & Frank, E. (2008). Which symptoms predict recurrence of depression in women treated with maintenance interpersonal psychotherapy? *Depression and Anxiety, 25*(12), 1060–1066. https://doi.org/10.1002/da.20467

Edwards, S. D. (2015). HeartMath: A positive psychology paradigm for promoting psychophysiological and global coherence. *Journal of Psychology in Africa, 25*(4), 367–374. https://doi.org/10.1080/14330237.2015.1078104

Ehlers, A., Mauchnik, J., & Handley, R. (2012). Reducing unwanted trauma memories by imaginal exposure or autobiographical memory elaboration: An analogue study of memory processes. *Journal of Behavior Therapy and Experimental Psychiatry, 43*, S67–S75. https://doi.org/10.1016/j.jbtep.2010.12.009

Flynn, M., & Rudolph, K. D. (2014). A prospective examination of emotional clarity, stress responses, and depressive symptoms during early adolescence. *The Journal of Early Adolescence, 34*(7), 923–939. https://doi.org/10.1177/0272431613513959

Fox, G. R., Kaplan, J., Damasio, H., & Damasio, A. (2015). Neural correlates of gratitude. *Frontiers in Psychology, 6*, 1491. https://doi.org/10.1177/0272431613513959

Gambin, M., & Sharp, C. (2018). The relations between empathy, guilt, shame and depression in inpatient adolescents. *Journal of Affective Disorders, 241*, 381–387. https://doi.org/10.1016/j.jad.2018.08.068

García-Toro, M., Ibarra, O., Gili, M., Serrano, M. J., Oliván, B., Vicens, E., & Roca, M. (2012). Four hygienic-dietary recommendations as add-on treatment in depression: A randomized-controlled trial. *Journal of Affective Disorders, 140*(2), 200–203. https://doi.org/10.1016/j.jad.2012.03.031

Gendlin, E. T. (1969). Focusing. *Psychotherapy: Theory, Research & Practice, 6*(1), 4–15. https://doi.org/10.1037/h0088716

Guendelman, S., Medeiros, S., & Rampes, H. (2017). Mindfulness and emotion regulation: Insights from neurobiological, psychological, and clinical studies. *Frontiers in Psychology, 8*, 220. https://doi.org/10.3389/fpsyg.2017.00220

Hofmann, S. G., & Hay, A. C. (2018). Rethinking avoidance: Toward a balanced approach to avoidance in treating anxiety disorders. *Journal of Anxiety Disorders, 55*, 14–21. https://doi.org/10.1016/j.janxdis.2018.03.004

Hopper, S. I., Murray, S. L., Ferrara, L. R., & Singleton, J. K. (2019). Effectiveness of diaphragmatic breathing for reducing physiological and psychological stress in adults: A quantitative systematic review. *JBI Database of Systematic Reviews and Implementation Reports, 17*(9), 1855–1876. https://doi.org/10.11124/JBISRIR-2017-003848

Iyadurai, L., Visser, R. M., Lau-Zhu, A., Porcheret, K., Horsch, A., Holmes, E. A., & James, E. L. (2019). Intrusive memories of trauma: A target for research bridging cognitive science and its clinical application. *Clinical Psychology Review, 69*, 67–82. https://doi.org/10.1016/j.cpr.2018.08.005

Jacka, F. N. (2017). Nutritional psychiatry: Where to next? *EBioMedicine, 17*, 24–29. https://doi.org/10.1016/j.ebiom.2017.02.020

Jacka, F. N., Mykletun, A., & Berk, M. (2012). Moving towards a population health approach to the primary prevention of common mental disorders. *BMC Medicine, 10*(1), 149. https://doi.org/10.1186/1741-7015-10-149

Jacka, F. N., Pasco, J. A., Mykletun, A., Williams, L. J., Hodge, A. M., O'Reilly, S. L., Nicholson, G. C., Kotowicz, M. A., Berk, M. (2010). Association of Western and traditional diets with depression and anxiety in women. *The American Journal of Psychiatry, 167*(3), 305–311. https://doi.org/10.1176/appi.ajp.2009.09060881

Jerath, R., Crawford, M. W., Barnes, V. A., & Harden, K. (2015). Self-regulation of breathing as a primary treatment of anxiety. *Applied Psychophysiology and Biofeedback, 40*(2), 107–115. https://doi.org/10.1007/s10484-015-9279-8

Keshet, H., Foa, E. B., & Gilboa-Schechtman, E. (2019, July). Women's self-perceptions in the aftermath of trauma: The role of trauma-centrality and trauma-type. *Psychological Trauma, 11*(5), 542–550. https://doi.org/10.1037/tra0000393

Knapen, J., Vancampfort, D., Moriën, Y., & Marchal, Y. (2015). Exercise therapy improves both mental and physical health in patients with major depression. *Disability and Rehabilitation, 37*(16), 1490–1495. https://doi.org/10.3109/09638288.2014.972579

Kop, W. J., Stein, P. K., Tracy, R. P., Barzilay, J. I., Schulz, R., & Gottdiener, J. S. (2010). Autonomic nervous system dysfunction and inflammation contribute to the increased cardiovascular mortality risk associated with depression. *Psychosomatic Medicine, 72*(7), 626. https://doi.org/10.1097/PSY.0b013e3181eadd2b

Kozlowska, K., Walker, P., McLean, L., & Carrive, P. (2015). Fear and the defense cascade: Clinical implications and management. *Harvard Review of Psychiatry, 23*(4), 263–287. https://doi.org/10.1097/HRP.0000000000000065

Kranzler, A., Young, J. F., Hankin, B. L., Abela, J. R. Z., Elias, M. J., & Selby, E. A. (2016). Emotional awareness: A transdiagnostic predictor of depression and anxiety for children and adolescents. *Journal of Clinical Child & Adolescent Psychology, 45*(3), 262–269. https://doi.org/10.1080/15374416.2014.987379

Kreibig, S. D. (2010). Autonomic nervous system activity in emotion: A review. *Biological Psychology*, *84*(3), 394–421. https://doi.org/10.1016/j.biopsycho.2010.03.010

Kurtz, R. (1990). *Body-centered psychotherapy: The Hakomi Method: The integrated use of mindfulness, nonviolence and the body*. Liferhythm.

Lassale, C., Batty, G. D., Baghdadli, A., Jacka, F., Sánchez-Villegas, A., Kivimäki, M., & Akbaraly, T. (2019). Healthy dietary indices and risk of depressive outcomes: A systematic review and meta-analysis of observational studies. *Molecular Psychiatry*, *24*(7), 965–986. https://doi.org/10.1038/s41380-018-0237

Li, Y., Lv, M. R., Wei, Y. J., Sun, L., Zhang, J. X., Zhang, H. G., & Li, B. (2017). Dietary patterns and depression risk: A meta-analysis. *Psychiatry Research*, *253*, 373–382. https://doi.org/10.1016/j.psychres.2017.04.020

Lim, Y. H., Kim, H., Kim, J. H., Bae, S., Park, H. Y., & Hong, Y. C. (2012). Air pollution and symptoms of depression in elderly adults. *Environmental Health Perspectives*, *120*(7), 1023. https://doi.org/10.1289/ehp.1104100

Lopresti, A. L., Hood, S. D., & Drummond, P. D. (2013). A review of lifestyle factors that contribute to important pathways associated with major depression: Diet, sleep and exercise. *Journal of Affective Disorders 148*(1), 12–27. https://doi.org/10.1016/j.jad.2013.01.014

Luppino, F. S., de Wit, L. M., Bouvy, P. F., Stijnen, T., Cuijpers, P., Penninx, B.W., & Zitman, F. G. (2010). Overweight, obesity, and depression: A systematic review and meta-analysis of longitudinal studies. *Archives of General Psychiatry*, *67*(3), 220–229. https://doi.org/10.1001/archgenpsychiatry.2010.2

Maes, M., Fišar, Z., Medina, M., Scapagnini, G., Nowak, G., & Berk, M. (2012). New drug targets in depression: Inflammatory, cell-mediated immune, oxidative and nitrosative stress, mitochondrial, antioxidant, and neuroprogressive pathways. And new drug candidates—Nrf2 activators and GSK-3 inhibitors. *Inflammopharmacology*, *20*(3), 127–150. https://doi.org/10.1007/s10787-011-0111-7

Manber, R., Edinger, J. D., Gress, J. L., San Pedro-Salcedo, M. G., Kuo, T. F., & Kalista, T. (2008). Cognitive behavioral therapy for insomnia enhances depression outcome in patients with co-morbid major depressive disorder and insomnia. *Sleep*, *31*(4), 489–495. https://doi.org/10.1093/sleep/31.4.489

McCanlies, E. C., Sarkisian, K., Andrew, M. E., Burchfiel, C. M., & Violanti, J. M. (2017). Association of peritraumatic dissociation with symptoms of depression and posttraumatic stress disorder. *Psychological Trauma*, *9*(4), 479–484. https://doi.org/10.1037/tra0000215

McCraty, R., & Childre, D. (2004). The grateful heart: The psychophysiology of appreciation. In R. A. Emmons & M. E. McCullough (Eds.), *The psychology of gratitude* (pp. 230–255). Oxford University Press.

Minton, K., Ogden, P., & Pain, C. (2006). *Trauma and the body: A sensorimotor approach to psychotherapy (Norton Series on Interpersonal Neurobiology)*. W. W. Norton & Company.

Motivala, S. J., Levin, M. J., Oxman, M. N., & Irwin, M. R. (2006). Impairments in health functioning and sleep quality in older adults with a history of depression. *Journal of the American Geriatrics Society*, *54*(8), 1184–1191. https://doi.org/10.1111/j.1532-5415.2006.00819.x

Moylan, S., Eyre, H., Maes, M., Baune, B., Jacka, F., & Berk, M. (2013). Exercising the worry away: How inflammation, oxidative and nitrogen stress mediates the beneficial effect of physical activity on anxiety disorder symptoms and behaviours. *Neuroscience & Biobehavioral Reviews*, *37*(4), 573–584. https://doi.org/10.1016/j.neubiorev.2013.02.003

Mulkey, S. B., & du Plessis, A. J. (2019). Autonomic nervous system development and its impact on neuropsychiatric outcome. *Pediatric Research*, *85*(2), 120–126. https://doi.org/10.1038/s41390-018-0155-0

Ogden, P., & Fisher, J. (2015). *Sensorimotor Psychotherapy: Interventions for trauma and attachment (Norton Series on Interpersonal Neurobiology)*. W. W. Norton & Company.

Ogden, P., Minton, K., & Pain, C. (2006). *Trauma and the body: A sensorimotor approach to psychotherapy.* W. W. Norton & Company.
Opie, R. S., O'Neil, A., Itsiopoulos, C., & Jacka, F. N. (2015). The impact of whole-of-diet interventions on depression and anxiety: A systematic review of randomised controlled trials. *Public Health Nutrition, 18*(11), 2074–2093. https://doi.org/10.1017/S1368980014002614
Petrocchi, N., & Couyoumdjian, A. (2016). The impact of gratitude on depression and anxiety: The mediating role of criticizing, attacking, and reassuring the self. *Self and Identity, 15*(2), 191–205. https://doi.org/10.1080/15298868.2015.1095794
Phillips, W. T., Kiernan, M., & King, A. C. (2003). Physical activity as a nonpharmacological treatment for depression: A review. *Complementary Health Practice Review, 8*(2), 139–152. https://doi.org/10.1177/1076167502250792
Porges, S. W. (2001). The Polyvagal Theory: Phylogenetic substrates of a social nervous system. *International Journal of Psychophysiology, 42*(2), 123–146. https://doi.org/10.1016/s0167-8760(01)00162-3
Porges, S. W. (2005). The role of social engagement in attachment and bonding: A phylogenetic perspective. In C. S. Carter, L. Ahnert, K. E. Grossmann, S. B. Hrdy, M. E. Lamb, S. W. Porges, & N. Sachser (Eds.), *Attachment and bonding: A new synthesis* (pp. 33–54). Boston Review.
Porges, S. W. (2007). The polyvagal perspective. *Biological Psycholology, 74,* 116–143. https://doi.org/10.1016/j.biopsycho.2006.06.009
Porges, S. W. (2009). The Polyvagal Theory: New insights into adaptive reactions of the autonomic nervous system. *Cleveland Clinic Journal of Medicine, 76*(2), S86–90. https://doi.org/10.3949/ccjm.76.s2.17
Porges, S. W. (2011). *The Polyvagal Theory: Neurophysiological foundations of emotions, attachment, communication, and self-regulation (Norton Series on Interpersonal Neurobiology).* W. W. Norton & Company.
Porges, S. W., & Furman, S. A. (2011). The early development of the autonomic nervous system provides a neural platform for social behavior: A polyvagal perspective. *Infant and Child Development, 20*(1), 106–118. https://doi.org/10.1002/icd.688
Raboni, M. R., Alonso, F. F., Tufik, S., & Suchecki, D. (2014). Improvement of mood and sleep alterations in posttraumatic stress disorder patients by eye movement desensitization and reprocessing. *Frontiers in Behavioral Neuroscience, 8,* 209. https://doi.org/10.3389/fnbeh.2014.00209
Raboni, M. R., Tufik, S., & Suchecki, D. (2006). Treatment of PTSD by eye movement desensitization reprocessing (EMDR) improves sleep quality, quality of life, and perception of stress. *Annals of the New York Academy of Sciences, 1071,* 508–513. https://doi.org/10.1196/annals.1364.054
Raison, C. L., Capuron, L., & Miller, A. H. (2006). Cytokines sing the blues: Inflammation and the pathogenesis of depression. *Trends in Immunology, 27*(1), 24–31. https://doi.org/10.1016/j.it.2005.11.006
Rasch, B., & Born, J. (2013). About sleep's role in memory. *Physiological Reviews, 93*(2), 661–776. https://doi.org/10.1152/physrev.00032.2012
Rebar, A. L., Stanton, R., Geard, D., Short, C., Duncan, M. J., & Vandelanotte, C. (2015). A meta-meta-analysis of the effect of physical activity on depression and anxiety in non-clinical adult populations. *Health Psychology Review, 9*(3), 366–378. https://doi.org/10.1080/17437199.2015.1022901
Riemann, D., & Voderholzer, U. (2003). Primary insomnia: A risk factor to develop depression? *Journal of Affective Disorders, 76*(1), 255–259. https://doi.org/10.1016/s0165-0327(02)00072-1
Rimer, J., Dwan, K., Lawlor, D. A., Greig, C. A., McMurdo, M., Morley, W., & Mead, G. E. (2012). Exercise for depression. *The Cochrane Library, 7,* CD004366. https://doi.org/10.1002/14651858.CD004366.pub5
Risch, N., Herrell, R., Lehner, T., Liang, K. Y., Eaves, L., Hoh, J., Griem, A., Kovacs, M., Ott, J., & Merikangas, K. R. (2009). Interaction between the serotonin transporter gene (5-HTTLPR), stressful life events, and risk of depression: A meta-analysis. *JAMA, 301*(23), 2462–2471. https://doi.org/10.1001/jama.2009.878

Roelofs, K. (2017). Freeze for action: Neurobiological mechanisms in animal and human freezing. *Philosophical Transactions of the Royal Society B: Biological Sciences, 372*(1718), 20160206. https://doi.org/10.1098/rstb.2016.0206

Rosenbaum, S., Vancampfort, D., Steel, Z., Newby, J., Ward, P. B., & Stubbs, B. (2015). Physical activity in the treatment of post-traumatic stress disorder: A systematic review and meta-analysis. *Psychiatry Research, 230*(2), 130–136. https://doi.org/10.1016/j.psychres.2015.10.017

Roth, T. (2004) Insomnia as a risk factor for depression. *International Journal of Neuropsychopharmacology, 7*, S34–S35. https://doi.org/10.1016/j.psychres.2015.10.017

Russo, M. A., Santarelli, D. M., & O'Rourke, D. (2017). The physiological effects of slow breathing in the healthy human. *Breathe, 13*(4), 298–309. https://doi.org/10.1183/20734735.009817

Salters-Pedneault, K., Tull, M. T., & Roemer, L. (2004). The role of avoidance of emotional material in the anxiety disorders. *Applied and Preventive Psychology, 11*(2), 95–114. https://doi.org/10.1183/20734735.009817

Sánchez-Villegas, A., Delgado-Rodríguez, M., Alonso, A., Schlatter, J., Lahortiga, F., Serra Majem, L., Martínez-González, M. A. (2009). Association of the Mediterranean dietary pattern with the incidence of depression: The Seguimiento Universidad de Navarra/University of Navarra follow-up (SUN) cohort. *Archives of General Psychiatry, 66*(10), 1090–1098. https://doi.org/10.1001/archgenpsychiatry.2009.129

Sarris, J., Logan, A. C., Akbaraly, T. N., Amminger, G. P., Balanzá-Martínez, V., Freeman, M. P., Hibbeln, J., Matsuoka, Y., Mischoulon, D., Mizoue, T., Nanri, A., Nishi, D., Ramsey, D., Rucklidge, J., Sanchez-Villegas, A., Scholey, A., Su, K. P., Jacka, F.N., & International Society for Nutritional Psychiatry Research. (2015). Nutritional medicine as mainstream in psychiatry. *Lancet Psychiatry, 2*(3), 271–274. https://doi.org/10.1016/S2215-0366(14)00051-0

Sarris, J., Adrienne, O., Coulson, C. E., Schweitzer, I., & Berk, M. (2014). Lifestyle medicine for depression. *BMC Psychiatry, 14*(1), 107. http://www.biomedcentral.com/1471-244X/14/107

Sayers, W. M., Creswell J. D., & Taren A. (2015). The emerging neurobiology of mindfulness and emotion processing. In B. Ostafin, M. Robinson, & B. Meier (Eds.), *Handbook of mindfulness and self-regulation*. Springer Science+Business Media

Schiweck, C., Piette, D., Berckmans, D., Claes, S., & Vrieze, E. (2019). Heart rate and high frequency heart rate variability during stress as biomarker for clinical depression. A systematic review. *Psychological Medicine, 49*(2), 200–211. https://doi.org/10.1017/S0033291718001988

Serrano Ripoll, M. J., Oliván-Blázquez, B., Vicens-Pons, E., Roca, M., Gili, M., Leiva, A., García-Campayo, J., Demarzo, M. P., & García-Toro, M. (2015). Lifestyle change recommendations in major depression: Do they work? *Journal of Affective Disorders, 183*, 221–228. https://doi.org/10.1016/j.jad.2015.04.059

Shapiro, F. (2000). *EMDR: Desensibilizzazione e Rielaborazione attraverso movimenti oculari.* McGraw-Hill Editore.

Shapiro, F. (2014). The role of eye movement desensitization and reprocessing (EMDR) therapy in medicine: Addressing the psychological and physical symptoms stemming from adverse life experiences. *The Permanente Journal, 18*(1), 71–77. https://doi.org/10.7812/TPP/13-098

Shapiro, F. (2018). *Eye movement desensitization and reprocessing (EMDR) therapy: Basic principles, protocols, and procedures* (3rd ed.). Guilford Press.

Siegel, D. J. (1999). *The developing mind*. Guilford Press.

Stevenson, R. J. (2017). Psychological correlates of habitual diet in healthy adults. *Psychological Bulletin, 143*(1), 53. https://doi.org/10.1037/bul0000065

Taylor, D. J., Lichstein, K. L., Durrence, H. H., Reidel, B. W., & Bush, A. J. (2005). Epidemiology of insomnia, depression, and anxiety. *Sleep, 28*(11), 1457. https://doi.org/10.1093/sleep/28.11.1457

Van Praag, H. M. (2004). Can stress cause depression? *Progress in Neuro-Psychopharmacology and Biological Psychiatry, 28*(5), 891–907. https://doi.org/10.1016/j.pnpbp.2004.05.031

Watkins, P. C., Van Gelder, M., & Frias, A. (2009). Furthering the science of gratitude. In S. J. Lopez & C. R. Snyder (Eds.), *Oxford handbook of positive psychology* (2nd ed., pp. 437–445). Oxford University Press. https://doi.org/10.1093/oxfordhb/9780195187243.013.0041

Weinberg, M., & Gil, S. (2016). Trauma as an objective or subjective experience: The association between types of traumatic events, personality traits, subjective experience of the event, and posttraumatic symptoms. *Journal of Loss and Trauma, 21*(2), 137–146. https://doi.org/10.1080/15325024.2015.1011986

World Health Organization. (1992). *The ICD-10 classification of mental and behavioural disorders: Clinical descriptions and diagnostic guidelines.* World Health Organization. https://apps.who.int/iris/handle/10665/37958

Yap, M. B., Pilkington, P. D., Ryan, S. M., Kelly, C. M., & Jorm, A. F. (2014). Parenting strategies for reducing the risk of adolescent depression and anxiety disorders: A Delphi consensus study. *Journal of Affective Disorders, 156*, 67–75. https://doi.org/10.7717/peerj.3825

Yoshimura, S. M., & Berzins, K. (2017). Grateful experiences and expressions: The role of gratitude expressions in the link between gratitude experiences and well-being. *Review of Communication, 17*(2), 106–118. https://doi.org/10.1080/15358593.2017.1293836

4

Processing Episode Triggers With EMDR Therapy

Arne Hofmann

INTRODUCTION

When it is time to begin memory processing when treating depressive patients, it is usually best to focus on Episode Triggers first. The *Episode Trigger* is defined as *the stressful and sometimes traumatic event/s* that occur/s for most patients 1 or 2 months before the depressive episode starts. Most of these events are not classical traumatic events that include danger for one's life, but events that come from stressful interpersonal relationship events such as losses, separations, and humiliations.

This chapter describes some of the most common patterns of depressive reactions to such events. The use of the Symptom Event Map is encouraged to chart patients' negative events and their depressive episode(s) according to a timeline. This helps the patient to understand and the therapist to build a treatment strategy. The chapter also describes some of the different types of depression that can be identified on the Symptom Event Map.

DISTRESSING LIFE EXPERIENCES BECOME PATHOGENIC MEMORIES

A key to treating depressive disorders is processing distressing life events that have taken the form of pathogenic memories and are associated with patients' symptoms. The symptoms that these memories trigger do not lead in all cases to posttraumatic stress disorder (PTSD) or another clearly defined trauma-related disorder such as complex PTSD (C-PTSD), prolonged grief, or a dissociative disorder. Instead, some result in depressive disorders or anxiety disorders, or they remain merely a risk factor for a later occurrence for one of these disorders.

The clinical manifestation of pathogenic memories can take different forms. This clinical list illustrates the memories in ascending order according to their degree of complexity:

1. *Depressive Disorder Triggers:* These are pathogenic memories that trigger a depressive disorder, intrusive thoughts, or flashbacks and in many cases avoidance symptoms as well. Nearly all of these memories are described by patients as distressing when rated with the Subjective Units of Disturbance (SUD) during history taking. If the *International Classification of Diseases, Tenth Edition* (*ICD-10*), or the *Diagnostic and Statistical Manual of Mental Disorders, Fifth Edition* (*DSM-5*), Criterion A is met for a PTSD diagnosis, then determine whether patients should be given the diagnosis of a depressive episode with a comorbid PTSD or just a depressive episode. However, often, in many depressive patients, Criterion A is not met for the episode-triggering event. In most cases, these pathogenic memories and the experiences that trigger them have a clear time connection to the beginning of the depressive episode. We therefore call them *Episode Triggers*. Episode Triggers can usually be ascertained during history taking and are evident on the Symptom Event Map where they can be documented well.
2. *Early Childhood Memories:* These early childhood memories often are partially remembered and experienced as distressing when directly discussed during history taking. Patients can generally indicate the degree of distress well on the SUD scale. These memories do not lead to intrusive thoughts or flashbacks, as the connection between present reality and the past is partially or fully lost, or is triggering to only a small extent. In many of these cases, these memories are recalled only in a fragmentary manner at the beginning of treatment, but slowly become clearer over the course of treatment. This is especially the case when these experiences are less matters of clear experiences of violence or sexualized violence, but rather the various forms of distress that are associated with emotional violence, neglect, or other stressors of a severely dysfunctional family, as indicated in the Adverse Childhood Experience (ACE) scale. Pathogenic memories of this kind are first and foremost a risk factor for the later occurrence of many problems including depressive symptoms—they intensify depressive episodes and reduce the effectiveness of psychopharmacological or psychotherapeutic treatments.
3. *C-PTSD/Personality Disorder and Depression:* The strongest manifestation of pathogenic memories for depressive patients usually occurs with highly distressed people who have frequently had symptoms in childhood or adolescence and who—in most cases—have already received a diagnosis of C-PTSD or a personality disorder (e.g., borderline personality disorder). Many of these depressive patients have already suffered from earlier depressive episodes or suffer from chronic depression and/or a severe dissociative disorder. In many of these cases, the traumatic background of the severe depressive disorder is not recognized. The poor response to treatment, or the frequent relapses, or the fact that the depression has become chronic over the course of treatment nonetheless frequently indicates that these patients have more complex forms of depressive disorders, frequently those with a comorbid trauma-related disorder.

The World Health Organization (WHO) has adopted two new diagnoses in the new classification system of the upcoming *ICD-11* based on these pathogenic memories. The first of these is C-PTSD (6 B41). The *ICD-11* (WHO, 2022) definition is the following:

Complex post traumatic stress disorder (Complex PTSD) is a disorder that may develop following exposure to an event or series of events of an extremely threatening or horrific nature, most commonly prolonged or repetitive events from which escape is difficult or impossible (e.g., torture, slavery, genocide campaigns, prolonged domestic violence, repeated childhood sexual or physical abuse). All diagnostic requirements for PTSD are met. In addition, Complex PTSD is characterised by severe and persistent

1) problems in affect regulation;
2) beliefs about oneself as diminished, defeated or worthless, accompanied by feelings of shame, guilt or failure related to the traumatic event; and
3) difficulties in sustaining relationships and in feeling close to others.

These symptoms cause significant impairment in personal, family, social, educational, occupational or other important areas of functioning. (6B41)

The adoption of the new diagnosis of C-PTSD in the new international diagnostic manual took over 20 years and finally allows for a disorder-specific treatment approach for this usually difficult and chronic group of patients. In spite of all efforts of the international working group, the definition has still not completely captured the complexity of this disorder, as recent investigations show (Knefel et al., 2015). For example, the current description is lacking the frequent occurrence of sympathetic activation and body sensations, as well as the strong overlap with dissociative disorders and personality disorders.

The other expressions of pathogenic memories that frequently occur as comorbid with depression are the different types of severe dissociative disorders. These include Dissociative Identity Disorder (6B64 according to the *ICD-11*), as well as Partial Dissociative Identity Disorder (6B65). The disorders occur at about .5% in the general population and 5% in those receiving psychiatric care. At present, it is known that these disorders are diagnosed to a far too small degree, which makes treatment significantly more difficult (Gast et al., 2006).

Of the 60% of depressive patients who suffer from having comorbid diagnoses, complex traumatic disorders as well as severe dissociative disorders are the ones that most frequently impede or completely block therapeutic progress in the treatment of depression. This occurs especially when these comorbid trauma-related disorders are not recognized before the beginning of treating depression.

FIVE DIFFERENT CLINICAL PRESENTATIONS OF DEPRESSION

Even if the accumulation of pathogenic memories represents one of the strongest risk factors for the development of depressive disorders, individual depressive episodes are usually triggered by defined, distressing experiences. These defined distressing experiences can, in most cases, be identified, even if the patient suffers from a complex form of recurrent depressive episodes, each of which must be taken into account in eye movement desensitization and reprocessing (EMDR) therapy.

THE SINGLE DEPRESSIVE EPISODE

In many textbooks, the single depressive episode is typically displayed as shown in Figure 4.1.

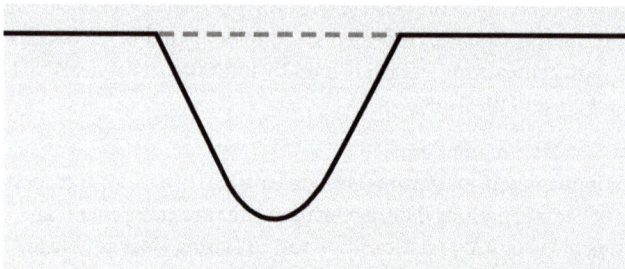

FIGURE 4.1. Depressive episode with complete remission in the typical portrayal of many educational texts.

Unipolar depression occurs in about 20% to 25% of depressive patients and responds very well to classic pharmacological and psychotherapeutic interventions in most cases. However, in the majority of these cases, a closer look shows that there is a distressing experience that can be identified before the beginning of the depressive episode. From the view of the Adaptive Information Processing (AIP) Model of EMDR therapy, the typical progression of this depression is illustrated in Figure 4.2.

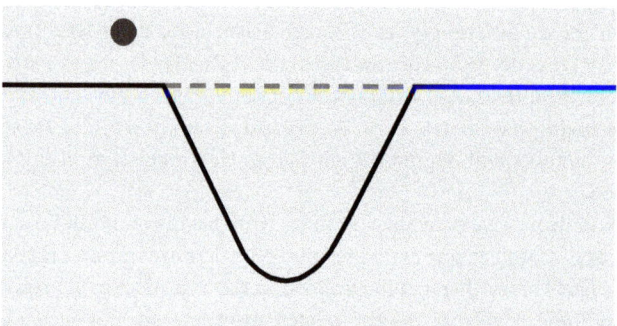

FIGURE 4.2. Depressive episode with complete remission from the perspective of the AIP Model.
AIP, Adaptive Information Processing.

In this case, the experience that triggered the depressive episode and the pathogenic memory resulting from it are represented by the dot. This form of representation is similar to the Symptom Event Map described in Chapter 2 and Chapter 14 for use in history taking in the DeprEnd manual.

Usually, single depressive episodes of this kind can be treated well with EMDR therapy. It is customary to find the Episode Trigger and then process this trigger completely with the help of the Standard EMDR Protocol. In most cases, patients experience swift relief. This progression is so typical that it can be supposed that the pathogenic memories not only trigger but also maintain the depressive episode.

In the second European Depression EMDR Network (EDEN) randomized controlled clinical trial (RCT) study that compares 16 sessions of EMDR therapy with 16 sessions of behavioral therapy (Ostacoli et al., 2018), there was a significant difference in both treatment groups at the end of therapy. Also, the EMDR therapy group showed that from the moment processing began with the memories associated with depression, the decrease in depressive symptoms ensued more rapidly. This change in the decrease in depressive symptoms, compared with the cognitive behavioral therapy (CBT) group, was the most significant finding of the study and shows the effectiveness of memory processing in the treatment of depressive symptoms.

Case Study 4.1

USING EMDR WITH ONE EPISODE TRIGGER TO TREAT AN ADULT FEMALE

A female managing director of a healthcare group in her late 50s came for therapy at the recommendation of her orthopedist who could not find any physical causes for her severe back pain. She suffered from a depressive mood, lack of motivation, and insomnia. She believed, "This professional situation isn't right for me." During history taking, nothing remarkable was noted. The diagnosis of moderate depression was made.

When asked what happened before the beginning of her depression, she reported that the group that owned the hospital was "taken over" by another healthcare group about a year ago. Since then, there has been a "new atmosphere" in how employees are managed. She was targeted as someone who was not "loyal to the party line" and was about to be replaced by the new owners. She began to notice that something was remiss when she was not invited to an important meeting about the future of the company and it hurt her very much.

In her EMDR therapy, the most distressing experience was chosen from the group of occurrences (cluster) around the company's takeover. She identified it as the phone call when she realized that she was not invited to the meeting. This was also the image she began with. The Subjective Units of Disturbance (SUD) was 7–8/10. The patient reported a guilty-feeling thought, "I am a failure." The experience was processed completely with EMDR. Two additional experiences about the company takeover were also processed completely. After this, residual symptoms remained when thinking about the building where the group's upper management is housed (trigger), as well as distress when she imagined the inaugural celebration for the new construction she had initiated (future template). Both were processed with the Standard EMDR Protocol and the distress disappeared completely. Subsequently, the patient regained her quality of life and strength. Her depression and her back pain disappeared completely, and she could sleep again. She could work again, but decided to leave management entirely and to start something completely new.

Alongside complete remission of a depressive episode, there is also the (more common) situation in which the patient only reaches a partial remission of their depressive symptoms. This is portrayed graphically in Figure 4.3.

From the perspective of EMDR therapy, the therapeutic approach remains the same. When there is a partial remission, we assume that patients have yet to resolve the symptoms

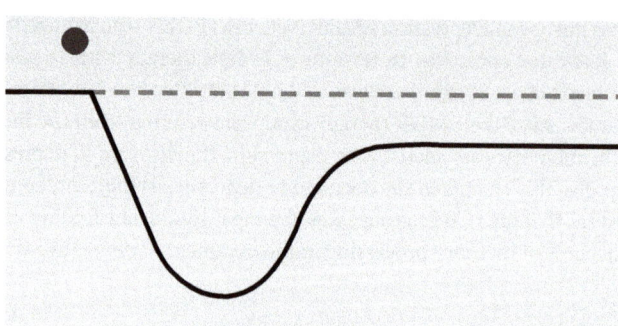

FIGURE 4.3. Depressive episode with partial remission.

triggered by the pathogenic memories over the course of treatment. Therefore, we focus primarily on reprocessing the Episode Trigger for the depressive episode. Afterward, we check to see if the depressive episode, including the remaining residual symptoms (dysthymia), have disappeared. If this is not the case, then we focus on present triggers that continue to maintain depression or risk factors that developed earlier and still have an effect (e.g., belief systems).

RECURRENT DEPRESSIVE EPISODES

The most frequent form of a depressive disorder is Recurrent Depression. From the perspective of the AIP Model of EMDR therapy, recurrent depressive episodes can be portrayed as in Figure 4.4.

With recurrent depressive episodes, relapses after the first episode can be frequent. Usually, the Episode Triggers for the first episodes are more distressing and more clearly recognizable than the triggers for later episodes. Nonetheless, clear stressors remain identifiable for many of the further episodes and also show continuing physiological issues, as reported with the SUD scale in history taking and the preparation of the Symptom Event Map.

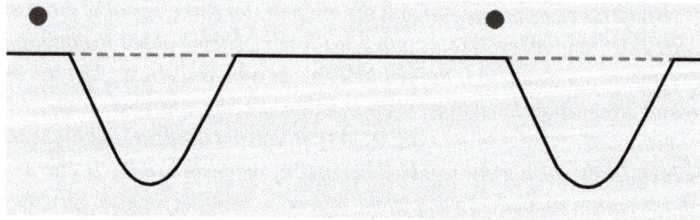

FIGURE 4.4. Recurrent depressive episodes with complete remission.

Treatment focuses on the Episode Triggers—as with depression with a single episode—and these triggers are processed with EMDR. For approximately 60% to 70% of patients, this is sufficient to resolve the current depressive episode. In the other cases, distressing belief systems or states associated with depression and suicidality are the focus, as is discussed in detail in the next chapters.

The practical question for what to do next for treatment is: Which Episode Trigger should we start with?

One important consideration when answering this question is to look for what we call a *Compensation Zone*. A Compensation Zone is a time when the patient last had a complete remission of their depressive symptoms. This Compensation Zone is easy to identify in the Symptom Event Map as the symptom line is along the dotted line of *no depression*. Finding the Compensation Zone is important because at that time of symptom remission it can be assumed that the patient's brain was capable of compensating for the distressing experiences that were experienced earlier. If such a Compensation Zone is found before the current episode, the first goal of treatment is to get the patient back into this compensated state without depressive symptoms. This means that the first targets for EMDR memory work are the stressful events that happened after the Compensation Zone. This is important as many depressive patients have traditionally high numbers of stressful and traumatic childhood events.

An additional reason to start with the current episode is the fact that patients who are currently in a depressive episode are also limited cognitively and in their energy level. It is good clinical practice to alleviate the current, most recent depressive episode as quickly as possible to facilitate quick progress for patients in their treatment. In some cases, the Compensation Zone is only found at an earlier point on this Symptom Event Map. If this is the case, the same logic applies and all episode triggering events that happened at the end and after the Compensation Zone are the first events to focus on with EMDR. Both observations, considered together, lead to the conclusion that it is reasonable for the majority of patients to relieve the current symptoms first and to reach a state of complete remission again as quickly as possible.

To this end, it is good practice to find the trigger for the current episode and then to identify the triggers of earlier episodes, especially if they are more distressing than the current episode, until reaching complete remission. Since we assume that the pathogenic memories of the Episode Triggers not only trigger but also maintain the depressive episodes, it is advised to identify and give priority to the processing of the last—and in some cases the most severe—Episode Trigger after the last complete remission.

In a next step, additional Episode Triggers, up until the last complete remission, can be processed. Generally, a marked improvement or remission of the current depressive episode will follow after this. With a noticeably relieved patient, it is of course easier in the following phases of therapy to process the remaining memories that trigger symptoms (intrusive thoughts, distressing belief systems, etc.).

Therapy is not finished at this point in time, even for patients who have reached a full remission. Therapy is now continued as a form of *relapse prevention*; and since the patients have already suffered relapses of their depressive symptoms, this phase of therapy is just as necessary as the first phase in which the current episode is resolved. These further steps of the EMDR DeprEnd manual will be detailed in the following chapters.

RECURRENT EPISODES WITH ADVERSE CHILDHOOD EXPERIENCES/ COMPLEX POSTTRAUMATIC STRESS DISORDER

In this type of recurrent depressive episode, one that frequently goes unrecognized, symptoms caused by stressors or trauma from early childhood occur in addition to the recurrence of depressive symptoms. Our experiences and clinical studies show that this type of depressive disorder does not respond well to pharmacological and psychotherapeutic treatment measures compared to other types of depression. Even when using EMDR therapy, this type seems to require a significantly higher number of EMDR treatment sessions to achieve an improvement in symptoms. In a clinical random sample, the number of EMDR treatment hours for this group of patients was about twice as much in order to reach the same relief of symptoms (measured by the Beck Depression Inventory, Second Edition [BDI-II]), as it was for other patients with recurrent depression. Since the majority of distressing memories that are the cause of this form occurred in childhood, this form can be represented typically as in Figure 4.5.

In the treatment of these patients, first the Episode Triggers and, if indicated, distressing belief systems or states associated with their depression are focused and processed with EMDR therapy. In some cases, treating belief systems or one of the states associated with the case of depression can be necessary before a (complete) processing of the Episode Trigger is possible. Generally, this situation can be recognized because the belief system and/or the Depressive/Suicidal States then are either dominant in the clinical foreground or significantly impede the processing of the Episode Trigger that is currently the target.

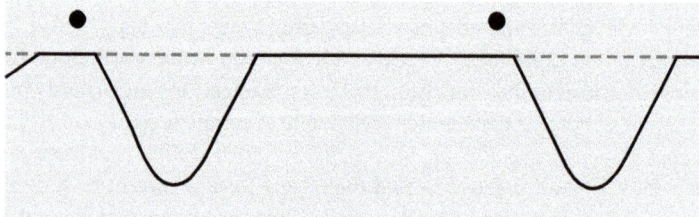

FIGURE 4.5. Recurrent depressive episodes with traumatization in childhood.

Distressing experiences in childhood can become apparent in very different ways in the context of depressive episodes. Symptoms range on a continuum from being completely symptom free (with or without amnesia) to a complete case of C-PTSD or a severe dissociative disorder. Distressing experiences of this kind occur in a spectrum ranging from ACE experiences to severe traumatic experiences such as physical violence or sexual assault (with PTSD as a disorder resulting from it). They are a risk factor for later depressive episodes, but can also be a complicating factor in the treatment of an acute depressive disorder.

In treating an acute depressive disorder, the distressing experiences that have a temporal connection to the beginning of the current episode (Episode Triggers) have priority over distressing childhood experiences. This is especially the case when there was a phase between the childhood experiences and the current depressive episode in which the patient's brain was in a position to compensate for the influence of the pathogenic memory (complete remission). A further indication is whether the reported childhood experience currently has active symptoms (intrusive thoughts, avoidance). If this is not the case, then they are of lower priority in the current treatment of the depressive episode. They should nonetheless also be processed with additional therapy in terms of relapse prevention, if it is the patient's desire.

The situation is different when distressing childhood experiences are active either as many intrusive thoughts or touchstone memories of a distressing belief system in the present.

In both of these cases, the corresponding childhood experiences become the focus of the treatment with equal priority to the Episode Triggers closer to the present. Here it is important to implement the appropriate EMDR protocol (like the Inverted Standard Protocol or Resource Activation), as well as to keep the associative channels limited while processing with EMDR, for greater control (like in EMD or EMDr, two more focused forms of EMDR memory processing). With the increasing complexity of childhood stressors, increasingly Depressive States also occur that must become the focus in treatment and be processed. This step in the DeprEnd Protocol receives its own chapter in this book (Chapter 6, Processing Depressive or Suicidal States With EMDR Therapy).

DOUBLE DEPRESSION WITH OR WITHOUT ADVERSE CHILDHOOD EXPERIENCES/COMPLEX POSTTRAUMATIC STRESS DISORDER

Double depression is a depressive episode that occurs in addition to chronic dysthymia. A typical progression is shown in Figure 4.6.

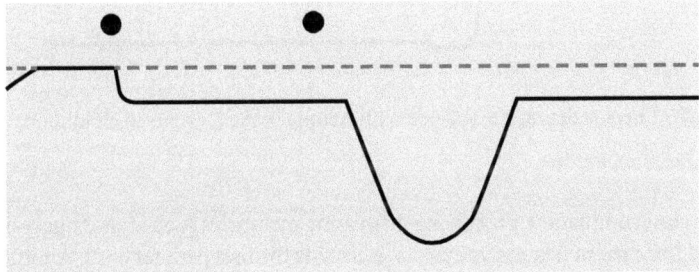

FIGURE 4.6. Depressive episode with chronic dysthymia and traumatization in childhood.

The distinction between this form and a recurrent episode with Adverse Childhood Experiences/Complex Posttraumatic Stress Disorder (ACE/C-PTSD) consists in the fact that a part of the patient has only partially or never been in complete remission since childhood. In addition, major depressive episodes occur. In this case, the treatment strategy is aimed at identifying the memories or memory complexes that are behind the majority of the present symptoms. These memories are then the focus of treatment. For example, it could be a memory of an event that caused a worsening of the depressive symptoms. A second possibility would be that the patient did indeed achieve a full remission of their childhood depression in the course of their development, but after a later depressive episode has not attained remission again and has remained dysthymic with recurrent major depressive episodes.

In treating a case of this kind, it is often possible to reach an improvement or resolution of the current symptoms by reprocessing the triggers for the first new depressive episode that occurred, after a phase of complete remission of the patient's childhood depression (Compensation Zone). When the childhood memories cannot be isolated during the processing of these memories, at first, with the use of the affect bridge, earlier active memories can be identified and then reprocessed.

In both cases, it is also possible to process these childhood memories for the purpose of relapse prevention in further treatment, if they had not come into focus during the processing of the present depressive episode.

CHRONIC DEPRESSION WITH OR WITHOUT ADVERSE CHILDHOOD EXPERIENCE/COMPLEX POSTTRAUMATIC STRESS DISORDER

Chronic depression is characterized by the fact that major depression has persisted for over 2 years. Chronic depression occurs in about 15% to 20% of all depressive disorders (Figure 4.7).

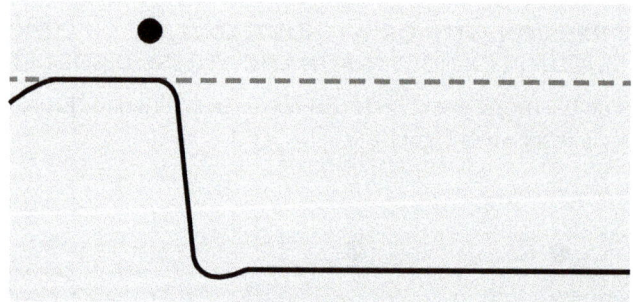

FIGURE 4.7. Chronic depressive episode with trauma or ACE events in childhood.
ACE, adverse childhood experience.

In this clinical situation, processing distressing memories such as the trigger or whatever exacerbated the current depressive episode is usually the best path forward. Another possibility, especially if no Compensation Zone is found, is to focus on active distressing childhood memories. The sequence of focusing can be very different here and is determined by the activity of each pathogenic memory, by the needs of the patient, and by questions regarding the setting (e.g., inpatient or outpatient treatment, interruptions in treatment due to crises, other medical treatments, vacation, etc.).

Case Study 4.2

USING EMDR WITH AN ADULT MALE DIAGNOSED WITH RECURRENT DEPRESSIVE DISORDER AND COMPLEX POSTTRAUMATIC STRESS DISORDER

A 54-year-old male patient was admitted to an inpatient trauma-specific treatment by his outpatient psychotherapist when his symptoms worsened. The diagnosis of recurrent depressive disorder, currently a moderately severe depressive episode that had persisted for 3 years, was made. The patient also received the diagnoses of Emotionally Unstable Personality Disorder and Complex Posttraumatic Stress Disorder. During the preliminary meeting, he said: "If this therapy does not help me now, I will kill myself."

History taking: *The patient was the second son (his brother was 4 years older) of a former SS officer and his wife. In his childhood and adolescence, a large portion of time was spent with his family outside of Europe. He was exposed not only to the gruesome war stories of his father but also the sadistic cruelty of his brother, who displayed behavioral problems. He was shamed by his whole family, due to his poor health. In early puberty, he began to abuse alcohol and drugs. By adolescence, he got involved with drug-related crime and prostitution, and despite his intelligence, he did not complete his secondary school degree. After completing an apprenticeship, he became self-employed in information technology (IT). Empowered by this success, he stopped using alcohol after going for detoxification treatment in his 40s. As a result of his emotional instability, he was hospitalized several times. His chronic depression—which occurred over 3 years—was a result of his professional difficulties with his client and inheritance conflicts after the death of his mother around the same time. Despite a great desire for it, the patient had never had a relationship with a woman.*

During his most recent clinical stay, the goal was to build resources and trust. After 2 weeks, EMDR therapy, three times a week, was begun. The main focus, at first, was the current Episode Trigger that was the difficulty he had in his workplace. The patient's mood showed a marked positive change after a few sessions. The next work was on negative belief systems ("I am worthless," "I am the scum of the earth," "I don't matter to anyone") which are connected to pathogenic memories of his childhood. The processing of experiences of violence in his childhood and adolescence followed. After 2 months of therapy, there was a noticeable improvement in his mental state. The last phase of therapy was devoted to the processing of the inheritance disputes and preparation for returning to professional life (trigger, future projection). The BDI-II decreased from 25 to 6. In the 1-year follow-up, he explained that he has been in a relationship with a woman for the first time for 5 months and that he was doing well, "like never before in my life."

Our experiences and the case examples show that in all five different ways that depressive disorders can present, even with the more complex forms of depression, many patients can still benefit from EMDR therapy. For many however the processing of depressive Episode Triggers is not enough. The processing of other pathogenic memories may be necessary to further improve the treatment results. These will be described in the following chapters.

REFERENCES

Gast, U., Rodewald, F., Hofmann, A., Mattheß, H., Nijenhuis, E., Reddemann, L., & Emrich, H. M. (2006). Die dissoziative Identitätsstörung – häufig fehldiagnostiziert. *Deutsches Ärzteblatt*, *103*(47), A3193–3200.

Knefel, M., Garvert, D. W., Cloitre, M., & Lueger-Schuster, B. (2015). Update to an evaluation of ICD-11 PTSD and complex PTSD criteria in a sample of adult survivors of child-hood institutional abuse by Knefel & Lueger-Schuster (2013): A latent profile analysis. *European Journal of Psychotraumatology*, *6*(1), Article 25290. https://doi.org/10.3402/ejpt.v6.25290

Ostacoli, L., Carletto, S., Cavallo, M., Baldomir-Gago, P., Di Lorenzo, G., Fernandez, I., Hase, M., Justo-Alonso, A., Lehnung, M., Migliaretti, G., Oliva, F., Pagani, M., Recarey-Eiris, S., Torta, R., Tumani, V., Gonzalez-Vazquez, A. I., & Hofmann, A. (2018). Comparison of eye movement desensitization reprocessing and cognitive behavioral therapy as adjunctive treatments for recurrent depression: The European Depression EMDR Network (EDEN) randomized controlled trial. *Frontiers in Psychology, 9*, 74. https://doi.org/10.3389/fpsyg.2018.00074

World Health Organization. (2022). *ICD-11 for Mortality and Morbidity Statistics* (Version: 02/2022). https://icd.who.int/browse11/l-m/en

5

Treating Belief Systems With EMDR Therapy

Maria Lehnung

INTRODUCTION

Treating belief systems with eye movement desensitization and reprocessing (EMDR) therapy is an important part of the DeprEnd Protocol. A second group of pathogenic memories that often need to be reprocessed in depressive patients are memories that create negative belief systems and negative self-concepts. Even though many depressive patients lose their depression after processing their Episode Triggers with EMDR, many still suffer from residual depressive symptoms caused by negative belief systems. In this chapter, we will introduce how to identify negative belief systems and two ways to identify specific memories that result in negative belief systems that need to be processed with EMDR.

PROCESSING NEGATIVE BELIEF SYSTEMS WITH EMDR THERAPY

There are depressive patients for whom it is not sufficient to process Episode Triggers in order to achieve a long-lasting improvement and remission of depression. For many of these patients, negative thoughts about themselves are at the center of their symptoms, because they are intrusive and encroach on everyday life. From an EMDR therapy perspective, we call them a belief system when these negative self-thoughts get in the way of daily functioning.

Case Study 5.1

USING EMDR THERAPY TO TREAT AN ADULT FEMALE'S DEPRESSIVE EPISODE WITH SOMATIC SYMPTOMS

Ms. Grund came to therapy due to a depressive episode with somatic symptoms. I communicated to her how I treated depression with EMDR, and since she had already tried another form of therapy that did not change her symptoms, she decided to give it a try. We began by searching for the most current depressive Episode Trigger. Ms. Grund's depressive episode began after her mother drowned while swimming in the ocean several years ago.

We processed this Episode Trigger and Ms. Grund felt relieved and noted a decrease in her depressive symptoms. However, her irritability and strong reactivity remained connected to negative thoughts about herself as a person, such as "I am dumb" and "I am unimportant." We suspected that a belief system continued to maintain the depressive symptoms.

HISTORY OF OTHER SYSTEMS OF NEGATIVE BELIEF SYSTEMS/SCHEMA

Negative beliefs about oneself as a person, about others, and about the future can have a decisive part in developing and maintaining depressive symptoms. The most renowned supporters of this hypothesis were the founders of cognitive behavioral therapy, Albert Ellis and Aaron Beck. Beck was concerned particularly with the etiology and the treatment of depression. In his opinion, depression has its beginnings in patterns of thought that the affected person has developed about themselves, the world, and the future: a negative self-image, negative interpretations of life experiences, and a nihilistic view of the future. Logical mistakes, such as arbitrary inferences or selective abstraction, underlie these negative patterns or negative schemata, as Beck called them. These logical mistakes manifest in *automatic thoughts* and *dysfunctional assumptions* (Beck, 1967).

In the 1970s, Aaron Beck's view of depression and its causes were revolutionary at the time of his first publication. Prior to this discovery, behavioral therapy with the focus on visible behavior was in fashion and no meaning had been assigned to cognitive processing. Subsequently, cognitive behavioral therapy became increasingly established and found its way into the mainstream of the theory and practice of psychotherapy, with Aaron Beck as its most prominent proponent.

The treatment approach in cognitive behavioral therapy is cognitive restructuring: a change in the patterns of thought that are considered the cause of the depressive disorder. Socratic dialogue is used to assist in changing the client's thought. This is a typical *top-down* approach that begins with identifying the patient's overall pattern of thoughts. Then an intervention is made to change the thought pattern, resulting in a transformation of the total structure.

Beck's student Jeffrey Young further developed and changed this approach with his schema therapy. From the background of his own clinical experience, he noticed that many chronically impaired subjects could not achieve long-term results with a cognitive approach alone. He also noticed that his patients thought and felt in certain patterns or *schemata*. He described them as *lifetraps* in his book, *Reinventing Your Life* (Young & Klosko, 1993).

Generally, these, early, maladaptive schema occur in childhood or adolescence, when core needs, such as attachment, protection, safety, or autonomy, are not sufficiently fulfilled. The schemata contain memories, cognitions, emotions, and bodily sensations and often result in dysfunctional behavior. Treatment requires interventions on different levels: Alongside cognitive interventions, similar to how they are used in cognitive behavioral therapy, emotion-focused interventions are implemented such as imagination exercises, dialogues with imagined images, and chair work, with the goal of helping the patient have an emotionally correcting experience, sometimes called *imagery rescripting*.

Schema therapy departs from a pure top-down approach by searching for old memories via affect bridges and attempts to change these through imaginative exercises and dialogue with images from the imagination. In this way, it integrates a top-down approach with a bottom-up approach, and helps change present symptoms and patterns of experience through work on these early memories. Through the integration of these two approaches, schema therapy provides a much broader, more eclectic framework, combining elements of cognitive behavioral therapy with those of attachment theory, Gestalt therapy, and constructivism.

NEGATIVE BELIEF SYSTEMS AND EMDR

Viewed in light of EMDR therapy, it is interesting that maladaptive schemata contain memories. For if a maladaptive schema—a negative belief system—contains memories, or is perhaps based on them, could it potentially be understood in the Adaptive Information Processing (AIP) Model? Then, correspondingly modified?

The AIP Model provides how the EMDR therapy approach addresses the etiology and treatment of mental disorders; it assumes that insufficiently or dysfunctionally processed experiences are the cause of mental disorders and are called pathogenic memories (Centonze et al., 2005; Hase et al., 2017). Pathogenic memories have the following attributes: implicitly stored, intrusive thoughts, easily triggered, and the cause of a distorted perspective of the future. Behind a given belief system, there can be a single, or possibly groups of, pathogenic memories that activate these beliefs. From the perspective of the AIP Model, it is the pathogenic memories that cause the negative cognitions.

The EMDR treatment of these memories or memory networks consists of activating a memory and its elements, and then performing bilateral stimulation. Through activation and stimulation, a spontaneous and creative process with its own dynamic begins that positively influences the patients' thinking about themselves and their expectations for the future. The AIP Model generates a radical bottom-up approach. Without processing the memories that had up until then been dysfunctionally processed, there is no adaptive change in the symptoms (including cognitive ones).

NEGATIVE BELIEF SYSTEMS, EMDR THERAPY, AND DEPRESSIVE PATIENTS

As mentioned, dysfunctionally processed experiences that underlie the negative belief system of our depressive patients are usually stored as implicit memories. They are frequently not reported spontaneously. But they are easily triggered and the affected people suffer from intrusions, particularly from cognitive intrusions. However, in contrast to posttraumatic stress disorder (PTSD) patients, the intrusions of depressive patients are *intrusive fragments* of unremarkable events with a strong theme of negative self-worth. Here, sentences appear such as, *You can't do it anyway, You are a loser, You are not worthy*. The experiences that underlie these are rarely reported spontaneously, rarely appear in a listing of traumatic memories or an EMDR trauma map or a map of distressing life experiences, and rarely meet the standard of a trauma in terms of the *Diagnostic and Statistical Manual of Mental Disorders*, Fifth Edition (*DSM-5*; American Psychiatric Association, 2013), Criterion A for PTSD. Nonetheless, at play are key pathogenic memories that *prove* negative belief systems. The negative belief systems are dysfunctionally processed early memories usually of a nontraumatic character that maintain a strong negative self-belief in the present, project this negative belief into the future, and contribute to the persistence of depression (Figure 5.1).

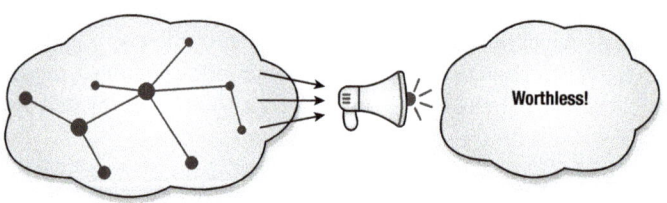

FIGURE 5.1. Networks of pathogenic memories as a cause of negative beliefs.

When we treat these belief systems with EMDR, it can lead to an improvement or lasting remission of depressive symptoms.

Since these memories are often implicit and rarely reported spontaneously, how do we find a negative belief system with its corresponding memories? First, there are indications of the existence and significance of a negative belief system inherent in the EMDR procedure itself. For example, when we are working on an Episode Trigger with EMDR but the Subjective Units of Disturbance (SUD) do not reach zero, Francine Shapiro refers to a *blocking belief* that is connected to a memory. She would ask her client: *What is preventing your SUD level from being a zero?* Often, the blocking negative belief system is uncovered. Or, when the patient is in the Installation Phase and the Validity of Cognition (VOC) does not reach seven: *What prevents your VOC from reaching seven?* Again, the blocking negative belief system is often elicited. Shapiro starts from the assumption that this *blocking belief* impedes further progress in the therapeutic process (Shapiro, 1995, 2001, 2018).

In addition, there are other indications that there are relevant belief systems blocking the EMDR process; for example, by means of symbols.

Case Study 5.2

USING EMDR THERAPY WITH AN ADULT MALE WITH A POWERFUL NEGATIVE BELIEF

Mr. Jens Müller, a banker whose career failed after a financial crisis and who was severely depressive today, came for EMDR therapy after a hospital stay. First, we worked on the

Chapter 5 Treating Belief Systems With EMDR Therapy

Episode Trigger, namely, the situation in which his employment was terminated. The negative cognition is "I am a failure," the feeling associated with it is powerlessness, and the SUD of nine was felt in his heart. In the process, a stone appeared early on: It was an angular, red stone, and his heart did not know how to get free. It then became clear that the stone was "always" there, and with some effort, we could put it away in a safe. Now it became clear that the "stone" was part of a touchstone memory that was a symbol for the belief system of "I am a loser." Later on in treatment, we returned to this stone, brought it into focus, and were able to uncover the touchstone memory that was hiding there.

Here is how to work on belief systems with EMDR therapy.

In the next session, we focused on the stone. The stone was associated with grief, and the SUD equaled eight and was felt in the throat and the upper body. Mr. Müller was then asked to drift back into the past with this emotion and this bodily feeling. Two memories emerged that had to do with being abandoned; we decided to focus on the one that occurred earlier in time at age 5 when he was sent to Norderney, an island in northern Germany, for treatment. The worst image is "When I was put on the train," the negative cognition was "I am abandoned," the positive cognition was "I belong," the feeling was grief, and the SUD equaled nine and was felt in the heart and the head.

While reprocessing, the patient relived the childhood pain, the feeling of being helpless, and impotent fury. When the process threatened to get stuck, the patient asked if he could take "big Jens" along as a response to the question of what could help him. The adult could speak with the child; the child felt warm and fuzzy. During this process, the two made an agreement with each other. After this, the distress could dissipate completely. The positive cognition was now "I am safe" and it felt true. After we processed the second situation that was associated with the stone, the patient began to emerge from his depression. He began to get involved with volunteering, started applying for jobs again, and said about himself: "I'm returning to life again."

Sometimes, signs of belief systems and the dysfunctional memories that underlie them appear in dreams.

Case Study 5.3

TREATING AN ADULT MALE WHOSE NEGATIVE BELIEF IS "I AM IN DANGER"

Mr. Petersen was suffering from depression and anxiety. Along with a lack of motivation, he experienced a feeling of inner unrest, that then turned into fear and panic, often the fear of dying—without any physical evidence. After we processed the Episode Trigger of his mother's suicide and he had had a positive experience of EMDR, a few days later he had a dream of a threatening situation with his father. He said that he had a good relationship with his father, but there was a situation when he was a small

> boy where he had had the impression that his father wanted to beat him to death. This fear of death that he had at that time still accompanied him today. In this case, the negative belief system was "I am in danger." Because this belief system arose with roots in a childhood traumatic experience, we processed the situation that appeared in the dream with EMDR.
>
> It was a situation in which he did something stupid as a child. The worst image was the moment in which he begged his father for his life. The negative cognition was "I'm going to die." The positive cognition was "I survived it," the VOC equaled 2–3/7. The feeling associated with it was fear of death, and the SUD equaled 8–9. Using the target from the dream was successful and the patient felt less tense and calmer in his body. In the end, he saw the situation from the outside now and said it did not bother him anymore. The SUD decreased to zero, the positive cognition "I'm alive" felt true. After the session, a new image emerged that was more positive and the patient's symptoms dissipated more and more. At the end of therapy, they remitted completely.

An additional clear indication of the existence of a negative belief system is the above-mentioned phenomenon of cognitive intrusions. If these interfere with the client's everyday life in their nature, strength, and frequency, we can assume that we are dealing with a belief system in need of treatment.

Case Study 5.4

TREATING AN ADULT FEMALE WITH EMDR THERAPY WITH COGNITIVE INTRUSIONS

> Ms. Clark had suffered for 22 years from severe, recurrent depressive episodes. The episodes occurred every 1.5 to 2 years and last year, on average, every 3 to 8 months. All depressive episodes were accompanied by the thoughts "I am wrong" and "I can't make it right." Ms. Clark told me that this had been happening as far back as she could remember. She associated it with her mother, whom she remembered hated her from the very beginning, never wanted to have her, and always signaled to her "You are wrong."

When we have this type of belief system, we have a specific process in DeprEnd to detect it, get to the bottom of it, and treat it. First, we look at the core statement that constitutes the negative belief system, such as the statements *I am wrong, I am unlikeable,* or *I am unimportant*. These negative thoughts can be deeply embedded in our neural networks and are often triggered. We search for the pathogenic network behind it, as these memories can be deeply entrenched in the limbic system.

Our first way to activate the memory network behind the belief system is cognitively. We ask the clients about the experiences in their life that prove the statement is true and ask how strong on a scale from 0 to 10, where zero is no proof and 10 means the memory is the strongest proof that the memory is true, how strong is the proof (de Jongh et al., 2010). Already, here, we begin to get an understanding of the belief systems. To completely understand the memory network behind the belief system and before working on these incidents with EMDR, we activate the second strategy and address the affected side connected to this belief system by focusing on an everyday situation in which the belief is active. Then, we use an affect bridge to let the client drift back into the past to the situation that is associated with this emotion, this bodily feeling, and perhaps also those words. The situation that appears is called a *touchstone memory*: It is the first memory of this negative belief system. If we process it, we open up the system in order to introduce an adaptive change to it (Figure 5.2).

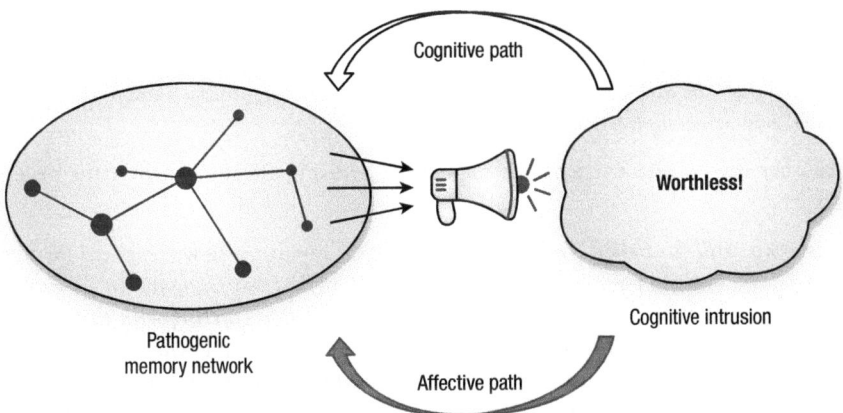

FIGURE 5.2. Two ways to find the memory network behind the belief system.

During the treatment process, we first process the touchstone memory with EMDR. In spite of its significance for the negative belief system, this old memory can usually be processed very well. Afterward, it becomes clear that the negative belief system has already begun to weaken. We can test this by asking about the strength/validity of the previous proof memories; often, their validity has decreased. Single proof memories that continue to have a high validity are subsequently processed with EMDR as well.

Case Study 5.5

TREATING AN ADULT FEMALE WITH EMDR THERAPY AND FINDING PROOF AND TOUCHSTONE MEMORIES

Ms. Grund came to therapy with symptoms of depression. As reported in Case Study 5.1, we processed the trigger of her depressive episode that was her mother's sudden death by drowning in the ocean. This helped Ms. Grund a great deal and her symptoms of depression decreased, but did not disappear. She still felt very reactive, irritable, and always had the feeling that she was unimportant. We identified this as a negative belief system and agreed to work with it.

Here is how to find proof memories:

First, we looked for proof memories by asking which memories "proved" to her "I am dumb" (or that the negative belief is correct). Ms. Grund had a number of proof memories from her time in school that felt distressing and humiliating and were still so present that we agreed to reprocess them. The worst image was when she stood in front of the class and was humiliated. The negative cognition was "I am dumb," accompanied by massive shame: The SUD equaled ten and meant that the incident was experienced today at a maximum level of distress when it was called up and triggered. In a very emotional process, we succeeded in reprocessing this memory completely. The distress disappeared, the SUD decreased to zero, and the positive cognition, "I am fine the way I am," now felt completely correct and true.

Another way to find a touchstone memory is by using affect to uncover the belief system:

There was still the belief "I am unimportant" that remained so we searched for the touchstone in this memory network. We did this by first searching for an everyday situation in which the belief system was triggered. Then, starting with this situation, we used an affect bridge to float back to an earlier time when the negative belief with its corresponding emotions and bodily sensations occurred. We tried to find the earliest situation the patient could remember and this was the "touchstone memory." We also called this process our affective entrance to the touchstone memory (Figure 5.2).

It was easy for Ms. Grund to find an everyday situation in which the belief "I am unimportant" was active: It was a regularly occurring interaction with her husband where she felt ignored. As we focused on this situation, the accompanying negative thought was "I am unimportant," the positive cognition was "I am important," the VOC equaled 3, the feeling was rage, and the SUD equaled nine and was mostly felt in her stomach. She was asked to focus on the emotion, the bodily feeling, and the words "I am unimportant" of this incident and to drift back into the past to find an earlier time she had experienced these same modalities. She remembered a time when she was 5 years old and she ran away from home and hid behind the local church. Her negative cognition was "I am alone and unimportant," the positive cognition was "I am important." The SUD equaled ten and she felt it in her lower body.

This memory was a touchstone memory. This very early memory represented many other incidents from Ms. Grund's childhood, when her parents had their own business and no time for her; her grandparents were the only people who spent time with her. Frequently, this type of memory also indicated the beginning of a chain of distressing memories that led to the patient's later symptoms. The distress resolved for Ms. Grund, and she said that the positive cognition was almost 7. As we once again looked at the everyday situation with her husband afterward, in which the belief "I am unimportant" was active, the distress had also disappeared from that situation and the positive cognition "I am important" felt like a 7—completely true. After processing these proof memories and their touchstones, the depression remitted completely. The patient described being full of zest for life and was much more self-aware. The physical symptoms that were connected to her depressive episode also disappeared.

WORKING WITH THE BELIEF SYSTEM'S TRIGGERS

When we process a belief system with EMDR, an important question to consider is whether there are still triggers or situations in the present that could activate the belief system in the here and now. These situations must also be processed with EMDR in order to completely resolve the symptoms.

Case Study 5.6

WORKING ON BELIEF SYSTEM TRIGGERS WITH EMDR THERAPY WITH AN ADULT FEMALE

Ms. Wal—who had processed past memories and was doing markedly better—could still be triggered in the here and now in connection with her belief system "I am worthless." This meant that her depressive symptoms could occur again.

A current trigger was the fact that her children did not answer her letters and they had not had contact with her for a while. As we focused on this trigger, the worst image that appeared was "Katarina's [her daughter's] facial expression," an image she imagined. The words associated with it were "I am worthless and despised," the positive cognition was "I am valued and respected," the associated feeling was powerlessness, and the SUD equaled 7–8 and was felt in the stomach. In the process, the patient was able to gain a new perspective, "It really isn't about me as much as it is about my children." Positive memories of her children emerged, she could recognize their dismissive reaction as immaturity and therefore accepted it. Her distress resolved. Nonetheless, the positive cognition "I am valued and respected" did not feel true.

This is a phenomenon that we often see while working with depression and EMDR. When we are dealing with a belief system that frequently has persisted for one's whole life, positive cognitions do not feel true so quickly as we would expect in other contexts in EMDR. Therefore, some work also has to be done on the positive cognition itself. We do this by first focusing on the aspect of the positive cognition that already feels true.

In the case of Ms. Wal, "I am respected" did feel true and we installed this positive cognition with bilateral stimulation. Subsequently, we looked at the other aspect that did not yet feel true to see if there was a place in the body where it was perceived to be "a little true." By focusing on the bodily representation of the positive aspect and following this with slow bilateral stimulation, we achieved a positive change. It was worthwhile to proceed slowly and to give the patient time so that the positive cognition could develop in all of its aspects. At the end of this process, Ms. Wal said, "I believe we are at a 7 [meaning VOC equals 7], even if I looked skeptical because I could now say, 'I know that I am valued and respected.'" Finally, we asked her if she could imagine a situation in the future that could activate the old belief system once more, and processed this imagined situation as a future template.

An example of future-focused work of this sort is presented in the next section. There are, however, clients who made it clear to us that their belief system could no longer be activated after processing the experiences that underlay it and said, "I know that I am valued."

WHEN ONLY NEGATIVE BELIEF SYSTEMS ARE THE FOCUS OF TREATMENT

For some of our depressive patients, Episode Triggers can barely be determined. For them, the negative belief systems frequently are our focus from the outset. How do we tell? Some depressive patients suffer most from interactional problems. For example, they cannot say no, are always exploited because of this, and thus avoid every possible confrontation. The negative belief system would be "*I cannot defend myself,*" or "*I am at the mercy of others.*"

Case Study 5.7

TREATING AN ADULT FEMALE WITH EMDR THERAPY WITH THE FOCUS ON NEGATIVE BELIEF SYSTEMS

This is the case of Ms. Rod. She came to therapy with marked symptoms of depression and burnout. It became clear that many of her symptoms had their roots in the fact that she could not handle conflict. She could not say "no." Partners and employers exploited this. It quickly became clear that this was not because she lacked social skills; rather, there was a negative belief system underlying this lack: "I cannot defend myself," "I am at the mercy of others." The search for proof memories unearthed a long list of distressing occurrences from all stages of life. We also searched for a touchstone memory and worked using the affect bridge as described earlier.

We had Ms. Rod focus on a typical conflicted situation as it occurred in her everyday life: a situation with her partner in which she could not decide for herself. Then, we had her set aside the image of the situation in the present and asked her to float back with the associated bodily feeling and the words "I cannot defend myself." She was directed to drift back into the past in order to see where she could find a situation connected to this bodily feeling, this emotion, and these words. We quickly found something. A situation from her childhood appeared in which her father spanked the children with a wooden spoon. The worst image was his face. The negative cognition was "I am at his mercy." The positive cognition was "I am strong, I can defend myself." The VOC equaled 4, the feeling associated with the image and the negative cognition was fear. The SUD equaled eight. The patient felt this distress in her heart. During the EMDR process, in which the patient first remembered pain and experienced rage, peace and strength finally emerged. At the end, the distress dropped to zero. The positive cognition "I am strong and can defend myself" now felt true. We processed two additional, similar situations that were part of this memory cluster with this patient. She felt empowered on the inside and started caring more for herself and paid attention to not coming up short.

As always when working with EMDR, we also checked to see if the negative belief system could still be triggered in the future. It became apparent that it was important to work with a future template in this case, as well. Here, we focused on the fear of not being able to say no in the future and then ended up exhausted and depressed. The situation that she feared and that we worked with was that the patient now had a new job lined up after being unable to work for a long time. Her biggest fear was that her boss would exploit and overburden her and that she would not be able to stand up for herself. The negative cognition was once again "I cannot defend myself." The positive cognition was "I can take care of myself." During the work with the future template, fragments from her childhood emerged. Then we worked with the situation at present. In the process, joy emerged, then the patient saw a rose. The positive cognition was ultimately "I am safe." This felt completely true and Ms. Rod experienced an internal smile that stayed with her on her way home. In the following session, the patient said she had made a great deal of progress. She could now assert herself and that had improved her relationships.

She then began a new job as a branch manager, and she was also doing really well there. When we ended treatment, Ms. Rod left empowered, with a new feeling of self-esteem and with the awareness "I am strong, I am safe, I can take care of myself." The old, negative belief system that had accompanied her for four decades had served its purpose and had been reprocessed.

REFERENCES

American Psychiatric Association. (2013). *Diagnostic and statistical manual of mental disorders* (5th ed.). https://doi.org/10.1176/appi.books.9780890425596

Beck, A. T. (1967). *Cognitive therapy and the emotional disorders*. International Universities Press.

Centonze, D., Siracusano, A., Calabresi, P., & Bernardi, G. (2005). Removing pathogenic memories: A neurobiology of psychotherapy. *Molecular Psychiatry, 32*(2), 123–132. https://doi.org/10.1385/MN:32:2:123

de Jongh, A., ten Broeke, E., & Meijer, S. (2010). Two method approach: A case conceptualization model in the context of EMDR. *Journal of EMDR Practice and Research, 4*(1), 12–21. https://doi.org/10.1891/1933-3196.4.1.12

Hase, M., Balmaceda, U. M., Ostacoli, L., Liebermann, P., & Hofmann, A. (2017). The AIP model of EMDR therapy and pathogenic memories. *Frontiers in Psychology, 8*, 1578. https://doi.org/10.3389/fpsyg.2017.01578

Shapiro, F. (1995). *Eye movement desensitization and reprocessing: Basic principles, protocols and procedures* (1st ed.). Guilford Press.

Shapiro, F. (2001). *Eye movement desensitization and reprocessing: Basic principles, protocols and procedures* (2nd ed.). W. W. Norton & Company.

Shapiro, F. (2018). *Eye movement desensitization and reprocessing (EMDR) therapy. Basic principles, protocols and procedure* (3rd ed.). Guilford Press.

Young, J. E., & Klosko, J. S. (1993). *Reinventing your life*. Plume Books.

6

Processing Depressive or Suicidal States With EMDR Therapy

Michael Hase

INTRODUCTION

There are certain types of memories, such as those of being depressed or suicidal, that patients experienced earlier in their lives; however, when these memories come up in the present, it feels as if they are true in the present, but they really are not. It is confusing for both patients and therapists alike. Often these memories are accompanied by intense feelings in the body but are not accompanied by images or thoughts. Often, they are overlooked even though they are, in our observation, a risk factor for depressive relapse. Even though many of the patients treated with eye movement desensitization and reprocessing (EMDR) DeprEnd improve during the previously mentioned parts of the DeprEnd Protocol, they may take another major step forward after their Depressive and Suicidal States/memories are reprocessed. In this chapter, we explain how to identify these Depressive and Suicidal States and how to process them with EMDR therapy.

BODY MEMORIES OF INTENSE DEPRESSIVE AND SUICIDAL FEELINGS

Clinical experience shows that the severity of a depressive episode increases with the number of previous episodes. A Dutch working group was able to show that 283 patients in treatment with the diagnosis of recurrent depression also showed noticeable problems during remission. The number of previous episodes was correlated with a depressed mood and this in turn was predictive of an additional episode. The authors refer to this phenomenon as *emotional scarring* (van Rijsbergen et al., 2015).

At times, there are also reports of an apparent resistance to treatment: Antidepressants that had been used earlier appear to lose their effect. How can we explain these troubling observations? The Adaptive Information Processing (AIP) Model of EMDR therapy can help here. In terms of the AIP Model, the very powerful experience of a state of illness (the memory of the body feeling *being ill*) could also remain unprocessed and then continue to cause symptoms as a maladaptive, dysfunctionally stored memory. We already know this phenomenon from persisting triggers. The memories of a recent incident, where triggers remain active even after the processing of the main memory, are caused by a secondary network that needs to be processed with the 3-Pronged Protocol of the Standard EMDR Protocol, as part of the present. Similar experiences are also reported in working with patients with headaches. A longer exposure to pain appears to lead to the formation of a specific pain memory that is experienced as an actual headache but does not respond to treatment with a medication such as triptane. Reprocessing these *pain memories* reduces the number and intensity of headaches (Konuk et al., 2011). Side effects of a treatment medication could also become symptomatic in this way. This also changes after reprocessing, as was shown by the case series of the treatment of adolescent rheumatic patients who suffered from side effects of the medication when they were treated with methotrexate (Höfel et al., 2018).

REMEMBERING BEING "DEPRESSED" OR "SUICIDAL"

It could also be the case that memories of being *depressed* or *suicidal* become triggerable nodes of their own or form a secondary network. Here, the phenomenon of *resistance to treatment* becomes understandable. If the feeling of a depressive mood is a memory of an earlier state of being depressed, then another patho-mechanism would be at play—namely, the mechanism of a pathogenic memory (Hase et al., 2017)—and a pharmacological treatment is expected to have little effect here. In this respect, one can expect in the case of chronically recurrent depression with a long duration, that memories of being *depressed* or *suicidal* will come up later, even if the illness has already abated in its primary dynamic or the essential material has been reprocessed. This also implies that working on Depressive or Suicidal States must be placed later in the sequence of the protocol. The word *state* is a provisional working term that captures the character of the condition experienced by the patient. In the AIP Model, this would be understood, as said, as a memory network, though the identification of individual memories can become difficult after a long period of time. The often somatoform memories appear to flow into one another.

The use of the word *state* is not to be confused with the term *state* as it is used in ego state therapy. Such states as described by Federn and other authors usually have parts that are close to consciousness, that barely occur in the states we describe—except in the case of a severe dissociative disorder (Federn, 1952).

Clinical indications of Depressive or Suicidal States could be a transient worsening of mood of limited duration that the patient experiences as a relapse into depression and is connected with a high level of fear of a new episode. It seems that this can actually lead to new depressive episodes in terms of a vicious circle, such that there is an indication for reprocessing the states. Intrusive fragments of an earlier Suicidal State can also be indications of a state. This is typically experienced in an ego-dystonic matter and can cause great agitation. It goes without saying that the declaration of suicidal intentions with concrete plans and without the ability to negotiate a no-harm agreement would be an indication of

Chapter 6 Processing Depressive or Suicidal States With EMDR Therapy 123

another dynamic and an immediate reason to intervene and guarantee the patient's protection through appropriate measures.

DEPRESSIVE AND SUICIDAL STATES

After working with Episode Triggers and belief systems results in the patient's stabilization, memories of the experience of having depressive symptoms, being depressed, or experiencing suicidal tendencies can be identified and reprocessed. We start from the assumption that experiencing depressive symptoms or suicidal tendencies can lead to unprocessed pathogenic memories due to the high distress associated with such states. We have chosen the term *state* for this since our clinical observations correspond most closely with the conditions described by Horowitz in his book *States of Mind*. Horowitz describes a state as a repeated pattern of experience and behavior, that can be both verbal and nonverbal (Horowitz, 1979). The states that we describe in this chapter are nonverbal in the vast majority of cases and the affected persons experience them with a high degree of negative body sensations and neuro-vegetative symptoms. These states have a clear influence on the patients' behavior, and are accompanied with a high degree of psychological stress. From the perspective of the AIP Model, we understand these states as memory networks that represent an earlier Depressive State or Suicidal State. Clinically, we generally begin with the Depressive State and then proceed, if necessary, to the Suicidal State. When there are multiple memories that can be identified, a cluster strategy should be considered (e.g., target sequence: first, worst, last memory).

Reprocessing Suicidal States should only be carried out after symptoms have been relieved through previous memory work, active suicidal tendencies have ceased, there is a sound therapeutic relationship, and the patient is currently experiencing distress because they were previously suicidal or are afraid of being suicidal again.

Clinical Experiences and Example Cases

As said, when working with chronically recurrent depression that persists for a longer period of time, it can be expected that memories of being *depressed* or *suicidal* appear later, even if the illness has already abated in its primary dynamic or the essential material has been reprocessed. However, a case of depression with few episodes can also lead to a state if the experience of the illness was powerful enough and led to the formation of pathogenic memories. The experience of suicidal tendencies can also be highly distressing for the patient and lead to the formation of a node. This is the case particularly for the early stages of suicidal development during which the patient is still wrestling with the decision. It remains speculative whether the curious release and inner peace occurring shortly before the act after the patient has decided to commit suicide can contribute to the formation of a node and to a desire for suicide. This problem requires further observation.

In reprocessing the material, the process frequently remains within the same network, that is, just the memory of being depressed or suicidal is processed. However, there could be the development of affect bridges to earlier material that has not yet been processed. This is more likely to be the case when the work on the underlying networks (Episode Triggers and belief systems) was less comprehensive. If the material that appears does not overwhelm the patient's capacity for processing, it is often possible to gain insight into the connections in a way that provides the patient with relief at the end of the reprocessing.

Case Study 6.1

TREATING AN ADULT MALE FOR MONDAY MORNING DEPRESSION WITH EMDR THERAPY

A male patient, 53 years old at the time of treatment, experienced his second depressive episode, which improved considerably after antidepressive pharmacotherapy. In the context of EMDR therapy, which we conducted in an inpatient psychosomatic treatment, we reprocessed the trigger of this episode, a conversation with his boss that he experienced as humiliating. This led to considerable relief. Over the course of treatment, we identified and reprocessed touchstone memories for dysfunctional beliefs. The mood of the patient stabilized further. Nonetheless, he continued to experience in the morning a low point in mood and motivation that was more pronounced on Mondays than on other days of the week. Since this stood in contrast to the otherwise good developments and the accentuation on Mondays led to questions, we revisited the patient's history again, in light of the AIP Model. The patient remembered that his first realization of his current depression occurred on a Monday morning after getting up. The identifiable target memory was this Monday morning, in the bathroom. The visual fragment connected to this was the look of his sad face in the bathroom mirror. The cognition associated with it was "I have no control." This memory was associated with feelings of fear, anger, as well as frustration and had a Subjective Units of Disturbance (SUD) of eight. The memory decreased to a SUD of zero. After the processing, the "morning low" failed to reappear.

Case Study 6.2

TREATING AN ADULT MALE FOR A DEPRESSIVE STATE WITH EMDR THERAPY WHILE HE REMEMBERS SITTING ON THE SOFA

A 43-year-old male patient was in inpatient treatment due to his third diagnosed depressive episode. It can be assumed that there were already earlier depressive episodes, beginning in adolescence, which nevertheless remained undiagnosed or were not treated. In terms of his biography, the patient grew up as an only child in a family in which emotions were not often shown. His parents' livelihood determined completely what the family did and did not do. Despite this poverty of attachment figures, the patient found connections via a sports club. He participated in cycling races as an amateur athlete. This meant that, along with training in the club and the races on the weekend, he also would train for multiple hours during the week after school, even when temperatures were close to freezing. The patient completed his secondary school degree and enlisted afterward in the military to have a career as an officer. At the time of treatment, he was an officer and professional member of the military. He sought out contact with the opposite sex only later in life, but was in a steady relationship at the time of treatment. His social situation was strained by a deployment far from home. At the beginning of the depressive episode, he lived during the week in a commuter apartment. The patient opened up to his partner around the sixth month of his current depressive episode because his suicidal ideation became overwhelming and he felt obliged to reveal this to his partner. She facilitated making contact to get treatment. During the diagnostic process, it became clear that the patient had suffered through at least two depressive episodes without seeking help. Beliefs from his childhood persisted that made it impossible for him to show weakness or to reveal his suffering.

During inpatient treatment, we were able to identify and reprocess memories of Episode Triggers and touchstone memories for dysfunctional beliefs. The patient experienced a marked clinical improvement. However, he remained in a morose, depressive mood and had a feeling of energy loss, which stood in contrast to his engagement in his everyday routine of treatment.

As a result, we decided to attempt to process the Depressive State as it lasted for months and was agonizing for him. The patient could recall a memory as the worst experience: sitting on the sofa after his service, unable to put any plans of activity into action, alone and isolated from the life that he could see through the window. This situation usually ended in darkness as the patient could not pull himself together to turn on the light, until he forced himself to bed, where he ultimately was unable to sleep. This was accompanied by a strong fear that his partner would call him and would discover his suffering.

The image was the gaze out the window and a part of the sofa. The negative cognition was "I am a wuss." Feelings of grief, fear, and disappointment accompanied this memory, which was experienced with a subjective disturbance (SUD) of nine. This memory could be processed to a SUD of zero. The Validity of Cognition (VOC), in terms of the positive cognition "I have energy," rose to six. After the session, his condition improved noticeably.

Case Study 6.3

TREATING AN ADULT MALE'S SUICIDAL STATE FROM INTENSIVE CARE WITH EMDR THERAPY

A 45-year-old man is in acute psychiatric, inpatient care. He came into care due to driving drunk after a confrontation with his partner. He has recurrent depression with comorbid alcohol dependency. In childhood, the patient experienced physical violence as well as being humiliated by his father and mother. He had attempted suicide after a relationship ended. After stabilization and reprocessing of Episode Triggers, his mood improved. The patient then reported a very distressing dream with suicidal content. He was driving a car into a tree. The patient is capable of negotiating a no-harm agreement and his suicidal tendencies were ego-dystonic. Checking his memories resulted in a memory that was easily accessible of the earlier suicide attempt by overdosing on pills, and then became intrusive and distressing. In the EMDR session, the image of intensive care appears. The negative cognition is "It's my fault"; the positive cognition: "I will learn from it." Then, reprocessing followed during which three channels resolved. At the end of Phase 4, the SUD is at zero and the VOC equals seven. In the next session, the patient is stable without suicidal intentions.

Case Study 6.4

TREATING AN ADULT FEMALE'S SUICIDAL STATE WITH EMDR THERAPY WHILE FEELING PULLED ONTO THE TRAIN TRACKS

A 55-year-old female patient with recurrent depression made a search specifically for outpatient EMDR treatment since she hoped that this treatment would provide her with better results. She had her first episode at age 13 and then experienced 13 episodes afterward, usually in the spring. The episodes ceased with the birth of her first child but began again after the beginning of menopause. She had been in psychotherapy for years and managed her depression with citalopram. Currently, she was quite stable with medication. After diagnosis, stabilization, and preparation for reprocessing, three memories connected to the current and earlier episodes were processed successfully. The patient then requested work for her suicidal impulses, which occurred on a regular basis when she was on the platform in a subway station. She then experienced a pull that felt like it was dragging her across the rails in front of the approaching train. She had always been able to resist this pull. A memory of it was brought into focus (Image: "Train tracks—urge to kill myself" with an atmosphere of desperation and hopelessness and a SUD of eight) and it was reprocessed. During reprocessing, a memory (5–6 years old) appeared: The grandmother told the little child about the war and the losses the family suffered. The patient felt the same atmosphere of desperation and hopelessness now in relation to this memory. The memory could be reprocessed to a SUD of zero. At the end of the session, a positive image spontaneously appeared that symbolized safety for the patient. This short-term EMDR therapy ended after ten sessions, four of which were reprocessing sessions. At this point, the patient was in full remission. In a follow-up after 5 years, she remained in full remission. In situations of distress which would have caused suicidality earlier, the image of safety that developed at the end of reprocessing now appears.

REFERENCES

Federn, P. (1952). *Ego psychology and the psychoses.* Basic Books.

Hase, M., Balmaceda, U. M., Ostacoli, L., Liebermann, P., & Hofmann, A. (2017). The AIP Model of EMDR therapy and pathogenic memories. *Frontiers in Psychology, 8*, 1578. https://doi.org/10.3389/fpsyg.2017.01578

Höfel, L., Eppler, B., Storf, M., Schnöbel-Müller, E., Haas, J. P., & Hügle, B. (2018). Successful treatment of methotrexate intolerance in juvenile idiopathic arthritis using eye movement desensitization and reprocessing: Treatment protocol and preliminary results. *Pediatric Rheumatology Online Journal, 16*(1), Article 11. https://doi.org/10.1186/s12969-018-0228-y

Horowitz, M. (1979). *States of mind.* Plenum Medical Book Company.

Konuk, E., Epözdemir, H., Atçeken, S. H., Aydın, Y. E., & Yurtsever, A. (2011). EMDR treatment of migraine. *Journal of EMDR Practice and Research, 5*(4), 166–176. https://doi.org/10.1891/1933-3196.5.4.166

van Rijsbergen, G. D., Hollon, S. D., Elgersma, H. J., Kok, G. D., Dekker, J., Schene, A. H., & Bockting, C. L. H. (2015). Understanding emotion and emotional scarring in recurrent depression. *Comprehensive Psychiatry, 59*, 54–61. https://doi.org/10.1016/j.comppsych.2015.02.010

7

Relapse Prevention With EMDR Therapy

Maria Lehnung

INTRODUCTION

Relapse prevention is an essential part of the DeprEnd Protocol. Although it is a significant step forward when the current depressive episode is resolved and patients are completely in remission for their depressive symptoms, in most cases, especially in cases of recurrent depression, one additional step is very important—relapse prevention. This is most important to consider even with patients who achieved complete remission. We have observed that most of the risk factors for depressive relapse are residual pathogenic memories, persisting triggers, and potential future psychosocial situations; these are the types of memories and situations that are likely to trigger a depressive relapse and benefit from the use of the 3-Pronged Protocol of eye movement desensitization and reprocessing (EMDR) therapy. It is also helpful to install positive resources that support healthy functioning in patients' daily lives. This chapter identifies different starting points that can be used in a relapse prevention strategy to inoculate patients against depressive relapse.

Patients who continue to suffer severe depressive episodes may experience an improvement for a short time and then they become depressed again—so severely that they have to be treated in an inpatient facility. Psychiatrists refer to these patients as *revolving door patients*. They are often considered *hopeless cases*.

Relapse prevention is thus a very critical part of treating depression. In the classic therapeutic literature, relapses are mentioned quite rarely in the context of treatment or as an integral part of planning treatment. What might be the reason for this? Perhaps patients and therapists are so happy to have reached a reasonably good result in therapy that they are not even *able* to think about a relapse. Relapses, thus, often become a taboo topic in depression therapy. The DeprEnd Protocol, as a new therapeutic approach to the treatment of depressive disorders, does address this issue and attempts to ensure that this treatment has more long-lasting results. Relapse prevention is an important part of the DeprEnd Protocol.

Indeed, relapses of depressive disorders are well known in the academic literature on depression. Relapses occur frequently after depressive episodes, especially when the patient only partially improves and an episode has not fully resolved, as is the case of about 60% of classically treated patients with depression. The relapse rate after 2 years is statistically around 50%. In other words, depressive episodes are most often repeating incidents. This is made more difficult by the fact that, in most cases, every additional episode—that is, every relapse—is triggered by a smaller occurrence. This means that the threshold for triggering a new depressive episode is reached easily. Additionally, the depressive episode that follows an earlier one is generally more severe than the preceding one. In this way, relapses represent a problem that must be taken seriously in the treatment of depressive disorders, and a problem that is an essential part of the treatment plan.

RELAPSE PREVENTION AND THE ADAPTIVE INFORMATION PROCESSING MODEL

Relapse prevention begins during the treatment of depression itself. The goal is to reach as complete a remission as possible of the depressive episode. From clinical research, we know that incompletely remitted depressive episodes lead more quickly to new depressive episodes. In the case of a complete remission of a depressive episode, we assume that the brain has succeeded in integrating all important factors related to the etiology of the case of depression. It is crucial to work toward this goal and to ensure the complete remission of the current depressive episode.

As discussed already in the previous chapters, our research on the use of EMDR for depression has shown that EMDR has a decisive advantage over other processes in this regard. In previous studies comparing EMDR with treatment as usual (TAU), behavioral therapy or psychodynamic therapy (Hase et al., 2015; Hofmann et al., 2014; Ostacoli et al., 2018), the number of complete remissions was significantly higher for EMDR. These significant results suggest that EMDR displays a particular strength in helping patients' brains and internal systems adaptively reprocess the decisive factors that contribute to depression. It helps patients reprocess and integrate triggers, resulting in a complete remission of the depressive episode. In this regard, DeprEnd includes relapse prevention as a critical part of treatment to make the results of treatment more long-lasting and to improve patients' quality of life over time.

EMDR DeprEnd is a therapeutic approach that uses the Adaptive Information Processing (AIP) Model as its organizing principle (see Chapter 2). This contributes to making relapse prevention even easier. In DeprEnd, the work differs from other therapeutic modalities that often focus on coping with the present. Rather, with DeprEnd, we start with the assumption that Episode Triggers or dysfunctional memory networks bring about relapses. As long as these are active, the treatment of depression is incomplete.

EMDR therapy always works on the underlying networks that cause the disorder. In DeprEnd, we work first with the triggers of depressive episodes, as described earlier. We also work with the belief systems and—to the extent they are there—with Depressive or Suicidal States, as we have discussed in the previous chapter. We begin by first processing past occurrences, then triggers in the present, and finally anticipatory anxiety of the future with EMDR. While working with trauma networks in general, we also work first on what underlies the current depressive episode, what caused the depressive episode in the past, then on current triggers, and finally on things that could cause a new depressive episode in the future.

RELAPSE PREVENTION STEPS WITH EMDR THERAPY

STEP 1: WORKING WITH TRIGGERS

Francine Shapiro underlined the importance of the *3-Pronged Protocol* that contained not only the processing of the past, but also triggers in the present and the future. In DeprEnd, there is more to consider. Not only is it important to completely process Episode Triggers, it is important to process negative belief systems as well. Processing triggers is an important part of the DeprEnd treatment model and certainly a part of relapse prevention, since triggers occasionally become independent of the experience of the old memory. An old memory can thus be reprocessed but triggers can still lead to a new activation of this past experience. By *triggers,* we mean all stimuli, in the present, that could cause episodes and all situations that could lead to a new depressive relapse. Patients can frequently name these triggers. Often, they simply occur in everyday life, and patients identify these situations and are surprised that they have their depressive symptoms again.

Case Study 7.1

TREATING A CURRENT TRIGGER WITH EMDR THERAPY FOR AN ADULT FEMALE

Ms. Wal came to treatment severely depressed. She had no motivation at all, she was barely able to leave the house anymore, and suffered from many anxieties. Working together, we identified and processed the Episode Trigger and also processed her negative belief systems. In particular, we processed a large belief system about worthlessness. She was now doing much better. In fact, her depression was in remission. She enjoyed life once more, she could leave her house, and she found new employment. This employment gave meaning to her life. The next step was to ask the following question: Are there triggers in the present that could trigger this belief system again today? Recently, a situation cropped up, a difficult situation with her children who no longer had contact with her. Due to a severe illness, she wrote them a letter. She wanted to have contact with them again, as she said life can be so short. Unfortunately, her children did not answer. This experience, the strong rejection by her adult children, triggered her negative belief system, "I am worthless," once again. Therefore, we followed up with work on this trigger.

How to Work With Triggers in DeprEnd

How do we do this in a practical way? We do this by having the patient focus on the current situation, that is, we ask the patient to take a snapshot of the worst part of the experience.

Case Study 7.2

USING EMDR THERAPY TO ADDRESS A CURRENT TRIGGER FOR AN ADULT FEMALE

Ms. Wal imagined the face of her daughter and her look of disdain. The associated negative cognition was "I am worthless." The positive cognition was "I am valued," and the Validity of Cognition (VOC) was at a level two. The patient experienced a feeling of powerlessness in connection with the image and the negative cognition. The Subjective Units of Disturbance (SUD) was eight, and the patient felt it in her belly. Using bilateral stimulation, the patient learned that it was possible to gain distance from this experience. She developed a new perspective and could see that it was a shame that her children no longer had their mother, but that she herself could still live well, even without her adult children. The positive memories she had about her children continued to be of value. She became aware that it was her children's choice to have no contact and to not get in touch, but this said nothing about her own value. All of these insights developed spontaneously during the EMDR process. At the end of the EMDR therapy session, the patient said that she was a valuable person. She knew that she was valued and respected.

STEP 2: WORKING WITH PROJECTIONS INTO THE FUTURE

Relapse prevention in EMDR DeprEnd does not just mean working on triggers, as shown in Case Study 7.2. By thinking from an AIP perspective concerning the future, we can understand that because networks that cause depression—just like trauma networks—are projected into the future, they negatively influence the patient's expectation of the future, and thus represent an implicit risk factor for a relapse into depression. As a result, an important step in relapse prevention is working with negative projections or anticipatory anxiety of the future. EMDR therapy understands these future projections as another aspect of work with dysfunctionally stored memories. Negative projections into the future arise through dysfunctionally stored memories and negatively impact the present and the future.

In depression, anticipating the future plays a big role. The anticipatory fear of a new depressive episode is an ongoing concern. Potentially, the fear of a new depressive episode is a realistic concern for the therapist as well, but often not discussed. In DeprEnd, reprocessing anticipatory anxieties are an important component of the AIP Model. By reprocessing negatively imagined futures, in connection with depressive relapses, these relapses are actually no longer an issue. The result is that the internal experiences of patients shift, leaving them with an increased sense of their self-efficacy and positive feelings in their body. The negative material that was connected to the future makes room for the positive material, and patients' thinking in relation to the future changes. The EMDR process is much more than cognitive restructuring. The new experience transforms the patients' experience cognitively, emotionally, and in their body, and, when there is a more positive experience of the body, it enables a foundation for a positive experience in the future.

Working with anticipatory anxiety is indicated when patients experience the fear of a new depressive episode. For many patients, this fear is frightening. If the patient–therapist relationship is good, patients are free to express this and say, "*I am doing very well and my family also says that I've changed a lot, but I am afraid I could get really depressed again.*" The next target to focus on is the image that represents the worst part of getting depressed again now.

Case Study 7.3

WORKING WITH EMDR THERAPY FOR AN ADULT SOLDIER USING A FUTURE TEMPLATE AND DeprEnd

Mr. G was a soldier and presented for therapy with a severe depressive episode, during which he was suicidal and was hospitalized. Since then, the focus was on the Episode Triggers, the most negative belief systems he was suffering from, resulting in his doing much better. However, Mr. G was afraid that he could become depressed again. This provided the focus for the next target. His worst image was where he was sitting depressed on the edge of the bathtub and had the thought, "I don't want to live anymore." His positive cognition was: "I want to live." While focusing on this future image and his negative cognition, he felt desperation. His distress level was very high, the SUD was at nine and he felt the negative bodily feeling in his belly.

While reprocessing this anticipatory anxiety with bilateral stimulation, he had a strong emotional experience. Old memories, particularly those of the last depressive episode, appeared again. They were resolved, and at the conclusion of the session, Mr. G could say, "I want to live." The experience of this work was so lasting that Mr. G said a few sessions later that he was now doing really well. The fear of a new depressive episode had disappeared. A few sessions later, he said that he was doing so well that he did not need treatment any longer. After a few sessions, we were able to end therapy successfully. Mr. G's report after a 1-year follow-up showed that his treatment for a severe depressive episode was successful and he did not have any additional relapses.

This is just one of many examples that show that the work with negative future projections/anticipatory anxiety in the treatment of depressive disorders, in terms of relapse prevention, can be very successful.

Another form of future projection is the *positive future template*, also developed by Francine Shapiro. This concerns a positive projection into the future. Patients identify a challenging situation in the future and then envision the imagined future scene as they cope successfully in the future while holding in mind the positive cognition and feeling. If a distressing moment occurs during imagining the future situation, it is processed with additional sets of bilateral stimulation. At the end, patients should be able to imagine the challenging situation from beginning to end and feel effective and positive. Note that the experience of self-efficacy has an antidepressive effect that has been reported in the literature.

For DeprEnd, relapse prevention means processing triggers in the present that could lead to a negative experience and may become triggers for a new depressive episode or activate a negative belief system. Additionally, relapse prevention includes the building up of resources for specific situations, particularly for potential relapse situations. Furthermore, relapse prevention also means working with the anticipatory anxiety of the future, such as the fear of having another depressive episode. When this fear is conquered, patients can look positively into the future.

STEP 3: BUILDING UP SPECIFIC RESOURCES

Building up resources is a strategic part of DeprEnd in preventing relapses with depressive patients. The efficacy of positive resources and particularly the conscious availability of positive resources has been documented for a long time in the treatment of depression.

In DeprEnd, however, we go beyond the traditional approach. We establish not just general resources with patients, but also work on building up specific resources for difficult situations that could potentially trigger a depressive episode in the future. Here, a resource is a positive body state that is installed using bilateral stimulation that makes it easier to access when needed later. For this purpose, Hofmann's (2010) Absorption Technique, as well as Korn & Leeds's (2002) EMDR Resource Development and Installation (RDI) are used.

Overcoming difficult situations is important for many patients with depressive disorders. If they overcome difficult situations in everyday life, then they have a new experience of their own self-worth and self-efficacy. In order to reinforce this experience, the Hofmann's Absorption Technique is used. For a specific, difficult, and challenging situation, specific resources are installed. This *anchor* helps patients have a successful experience in the future in this situation, a fact that represents positive empowerment. Particularly for patients with recurrent depressive disorders, often small everyday situations make them feel like a failure and then lead to a new depressive episode. In order to overcome such a situation well, they need access to specific resources, abilities that make it easier to overcome this situation. In the Absorption Technique, therapists ask patients which three abilities patients would need to be able to handle this situation better. These resources are then activated and installed with bilateral stimulation.

Case Study 7.4

BUILDING UP RESOURCES USING DeprEnd WITH AN ADULT FEMALE

Ms. Gise came for treatment because of a severe recurrent depressive disorder—so severe that she could not leave her bed for weeks and was not able to go outside. After we processed the Episode Triggers and the traumatic memories, we worked on which abilities she would need to handle everyday situations, such as going shopping, effectively. The SUD for going shopping equaled nine. She noted that she would need courage, composure, and inner peace as her resources and they were installed using the Absorption Technique.

We began with courage and when asked if she remembered a situation in which she had felt courageous, she said there was a situation on a train that was installed with slow bilateral stimulation. During this process, it was important to make sure that the corresponding positive body state was activated. The second ability was composure and Ms. Gise had no memory of feeling composed, so I asked her if there were someone she knew who has composure and she named the wife of the restaurant owner whom she had worked for, named Jemin. Ms. Gise focused on Jemin and where she felt composure in her body when she thought about Jemin and installed this ability with slow bilateral stimulation. The ability of inner peace was found and installed similarly.

After the installation of the three abilities, Ms. Gise's distress reduced markedly while thinking about shopping and now she was ready to actually go shopping. This success was a big step forward for her self-esteem.

Building up resources can assist patients in other situations where they might need support, such as a difficult situation at work, where patients quickly feel misunderstood or bullied. Installing resources with EMDR includes accessing positive body states as a way to help her in difficult situations. Using these resources can help prevent relapses in the treatment of depression. By installing resources with bilateral stimulation, DeprEnd goes beyond cognitive restructuring and, in addition, includes more positive emotions and sensations in the body that form the foundation for positive experiences in the future.

STEP 4: WORKING WITH THE MEMORY OF DEPRESSIVE STATES

Part of relapse prevention is an active lifestyle that contains movement and other important factors. While therapists can encourage this, we have observed that patients who overcome their depressive episode via DeprEnd develop a more active lifestyle on their own. Sometimes, part of relapse prevention includes processing the memories of a Depressive State. As described earlier, Depressive States contain, above all, body states and the memories of body states that have occurred before. The memory of a Depressive State entails focusing on that specific depressive body state.

Case Study 7.5

RELAPSE PREVENTION WITH WORK ON A DEPRESSIVE BODY STATE WITH AN ADULT FEMALE

Ms. Miller came for therapy because of a severe depressive episode. We treated her using DeprEnd, with success. Afterward, she began working again, started doing many activities such as working out, and overall was doing very well. Nonetheless, she still stated that she was stressed by her memories of the difficult times she had during her psychiatric hospitalization. In order to process these memories thoroughly to prevent relapse, the focus was on the maladaptive, depressive body state feeling. The worst image was "the feeling of being in a black hole." The negative cognition is "I am at their mercy." The positive one was "I'm in control of it." The feeling is a strong sense of powerlessness, the SUD is eight, and she feels the feeling in her chest. Ms. Miller focused on this target. During the process, the desire to be done and not burdened with it anymore arose. Another channel emerged concerning the ability to say farewell to this Depressive State with the recognition, "It is past." There is now room for something new. Indeed, during this farewell, something like melancholy even appears. Ultimately, the situation can disappear, receding like waves going out to sea. In the next session, the patient says that the preceding session was helpful, but very strenuous. However, the image of sending the Depressive State away with the waves is something that has remained with her. Afterward and ever since, she has been sleeping well again. The nicest part about this, she reports, is the associated feeling of not being burdened. The pressure she felt is totally gone, just like the internal unrest. This unburdened feeling, she says, was something so special that she got a small tattoo of a butterfly because it represented to her being unburdened.

The adaptive self-healing system of the human being, which is so central to EMDR therapy, can also be seen at work here.

REFERENCES

Hase, M., Balmaceda, U. M., Hase, A., Lehnung, M., Tumani, V., Huchzermeier, C., & Hofmann, A. (2015). Eye movement desensitization and reprocessing (EMDR) therapy in the treatment of depression: A matched pairs study in an inpatient setting. *Brain and Behavior*, 5(6), Article e00342. https://doi.org/10.1002/brb3.342

Hofmann, A. (2010). The Absorption Technique. In M. Luber (Ed.), *Eye movement desensitization and reprocessing: EMDR scripted protocols. Special populations* (pp. 275–280). Springer Publishing Company.

Hofmann, A., Hilgers, A., Lehnung, M., Liebermann, P., Ostacoli, L., Schneider, W., & Hase, M. (2014). Eye movement desensitization and reprocessing as an adjunctive treatment of unipolar depression: A controlled study. *Journal of EMDR Practice and Research*, 8(3), 103–112. https://doi.org/10.1891/1933-3196.8.3.103

Korn, D. L., & Leeds, A. M. (2002). Preliminary evidence of efficacy for EMDR Resource Development and Installation in the stabilization phase of treatment of complex posttraumatic stress disorder. *Journal of Clinical Psychology*, 58(12), 1465–1487. https://doi.org/10.1002/jclp.10099

Ostacoli, L., Carletto, S., Cavallo, M., Baldomir-Gago, P., Di Lorenzo, G., Fernandez, I., Hase, M., Justo-Alonso, A., Lehnung, M., Migliaretti, G., Oliva, F., Pagani, M., Recarey-Eiris, S., Torta, R., Tumani, V., Gonzalez-Vazquez, A. I., & Hofmann, A. (2018). Comparison of eye movement desensitization reprocessing and cognitive behavioral therapy as adjunctive treatments for recurrent depression: The European Depression EMDR Network (EDEN) randomized controlled trial. *Frontiers in Psychology*, 9, Article 74. https://doi.org/10.3389/fpsyg.2018.00074

8

Comorbidity With Complex Trauma-Related Disorders and EMDR Therapy

Arne Hofmann, Susanne Altmeyer, and Visal Tumani

INTRODUCTION

About 60% of all depressive patients suffer from mental health comorbidities. In many cases, the comorbidity of these depressive patients is posttraumatic stress disorders (PTSDs), complex PTSD (C-PTSD), and/or moderate to severe dissociative disorders. While structured research in this patient group is still in its infancy, in this chapter we cover what we have learned by treating many of these complex patients. It is clear that the greater the complexity with which patients present, the more psychoeducation, resourcing, and eye movement desensitization and reprocessing (EMDR) memory reprocessing sessions are needed. Often, complex patients have faced years of treatment and are not diagnosed accurately. Those considered treatment resistant are often patients with a history of trauma/PTSD or a dissociative disorder. The first step for these patients is to help them understand their disorder and to stabilize them before any EMDR processing. We have observed that when these steps are taken, complex and dissociative patients make real progress with their trauma and then their depressive disorder.

THE IMPORTANCE OF UNDERSTANDING COMORBIDITY IN THE TREATMENT OF DEPRESSIVE PATIENTS

For a number of years, research has confirmed that depression often represents a disorder resulting from violence and physical abuse in childhood (Heim et al., 2004). Studies have also proved that depression is one of the most frequent disorders to arise as a consequence of sexual abuse in childhood (Chen et al., 2010). These correlations between sexual abuse, depression, and PTSDs (as well as other disorders) are also demonstrated in a number of other studies (Gilbert et al., 2009; Jumper, 1995).

Of patients with severe depression, 50% to 60% suffer from one or more comorbidities with other disorders such as trauma- and stressor-related disorders, and particularly PTSD. These comorbid disorders play an important role in how treatment proceeds. PTSD and C-PTSD are frequently found in the general population. In a representative sample in the United States, one of these two trauma-related disorders were found in 7.2% of the population (PTSD, 3.4%; C-PTSD, 3.8%; Cloitre et al., 2019). This is important since many patients with a comorbid trauma-related disorder have more severe symptoms and treatment attempts are less affective. Furthermore, they have an elevated risk of relapse after depressive symptoms have abated. This comorbidity is often not recognized during first treatments of a depressive episode and is therefore not treated.

One of the reasons that the correlations are frequently not immediately recognizable in history taking is because experiences of abuse are not always accessible to patients or are concealed due to shame. The fact that depressive patients have had traumatic experiences often becomes apparent only over the course of an outpatient or inpatient treatment. Depressive patients are sometimes treated for a long time without their trauma-related disorder being recognized and specifically treated. Correspondingly, many of these patients develop chronic conditions that are only recognized later during a hospital stay. Usually, these patients have recurrent or chronic depression, as we described in the chapter on Episode Triggers, or in some cases also dissociative depression.

DEPRESSION AND COMPLEX POSTTRAUMATIC STRESS DISORDER PATIENTS ARE LESS RESPONSIVE TO TREATMENT WHEN COMPARED TO OTHER DISORDERS

There are many questions surrounding depression and C-PTSD. We would like to pass along our knowledge, particularly from our experiences in a specialized unit for severely traumatized and depressive patients in a psychosomatic hospital, as well as our experiences from a psychiatric university hospital.

Numerous patients from both hospitals reported distressing childhood experiences when filling out the Adverse Childhood Experience (ACE) Questionnaire (Anda et al., 2006). From our clinical work, we can corroborate what other studies report: The more the symptomatology, the more exposure patients had to adverse experiences. For example, Witt, Brown, et al. (2019) and Witt, Sachser, et al. (2019), working with a representative German cohort, showed the risk of a later mental disorder significantly increased with the number of distressing childhood incidents. In the high-risk group (equal to four or more ACEs), the risk for depression increased 7.8 times, in addition to elevated risks for other disorders. In another study, Priebe et al. (2019) were able to show that a large number of traumatic events led to significantly higher symptoms of PTSD in a group of traumatized patients than was the case for isolated distressing experiences. At the same time, the success of treatment in the group with multiple experiences of trauma was markedly lower with the same amount of therapy. Alongside the dose-response relationship, in which increased traumatization leads to increased symptoms, there is also a dose-response effect concerning the lowered efficacy of therapeutic intervention. In sum, this leads to less treatment success for patients with higher distress. In practice, patients require a markedly higher dose of treatment to improve the effects of treatment. This lowered efficacy of otherwise effective treatment for depressive patients with an additional PTSD can also be confirmed for EMDR treatments. In a case series of over 130 patients who were admitted to a hospital with a depressive disorder, the group with a comorbid C-PTSD required a noticeably elevated dose of EMDR sessions during which traumatic memories also were processed to achieve a remission of depression. This was different than the case for patients without a comorbid PTSD. It appears that the trauma dose to which these patients were exposed resulted in a more complicated progression and the overall higher need for therapy.

The degree to which EMDR can have lasting success for chronic depressive disorders without C-PTSD (a number of patients had a classic PTSD diagnosis as a comorbidity) is demonstrated in an initial follow-up study of patients with a diagnosis of depression who were admitted to a psychosomatic specialty clinic for trauma-related disorders and EMDR (Gezeiten Haus Schloss Eichholz, near Cologne, Germany). Of the 39 patients who were questioned, a full remission of depressive symptoms (Beck Depression Inventory, Second Edition [BDI-II], under 12) had been achieved for 21 (53%) at the time they were released. In a follow-up that took place after 16 months on average, 23 (58.9%) of the patients indicated that they no longer suffered from symptoms of depression. Three of these 23 patients, however, spontaneously reported during the follow-up that they had considerable stress due to the coronavirus pandemic, without that triggering a depressive episode. These results are encouraging, despite the small sample size, particularly because they match the results of our up-to-now unpublished first small retrospective study with 10 patients, described in the introduction to this book. There, as well, three patients had reported considerable distress without becoming depressed again. The resilience for depressive relapses appears to have been increased through EMDR treatments for these patients. Of course, more studies are required to confirm these findings; however, as is in the case of our other studies, this is an indication of a trend that the treatment of depressive patients can be improved further by using EMDR therapy.

While there are no systematic research data for patients with depression and a comorbid C-PTSD, and the need for a high necessary dose of therapy and limited inpatient treatment times is well known, there are nonetheless a number of encouraging experiences that we would like to convey through case examples to support using EMDR therapy with this population. Since the clinical course and plans for treatment in this patient group are very diverse, here are a few examples.

Case Study 8.1

TREATING A RETIRED FEMALE TEACHER WITH COMORBID TRAUMA AND RECURRENT DEPRESSION WITH EMDR THERAPY

The 54-year-old patient, a teacher who retired early due to recurrent depression, was admitted to inpatient psychotrauma treatment because she experienced frequent flashbacks of abuse from her childhood over several weeks and these flashbacks could not be treated in outpatient therapy. The trigger, presumably, was the upcoming birth of her first grandchild. During her own pregnancy, birth, and postpartum with her own daughter, she experienced extreme distress and anxiety. This same daughter was about to give birth and was becoming severely ill.

Her first depressive phase occurred at the age of 44 when she became overwhelmed due to a situation at work. This was followed by several outpatient and inpatient treatments, until the diagnosis of C-PTSD was made 3 years ago and trauma-specific EMDR treatment began, which was helpful.

Due to the severe distress caused by the flashbacks of the abuse from childhood, and since the patient was well acquainted with EMDR, we began to lower the distress caused by the images through the titrated use of EMDR CIPOS over a short period of time. (EMDR CIPOS [Constant Installation of Present Orientation and Safety] is an EMDR technique developed by Jim Knipe that uses Resource Activation and short contacts with the traumatic material to help the patient reduce the stress when confronting the material.) Parallel to that, we used resource-strengthening EMDR techniques (e.g., Absorption Technique) and then used the Standard EMDR Protocol for pathogenic memories related to the flashbacks. After about 2 weeks, the patient experienced significant relief and we agreed to process next the traumatic period associated with the birth of her daughter. This phase was very intense and energy sapping for the patient, and it took nearly 4 weeks until she experienced significant relief. In reprocessing, we used many affect bridges to access her earlier childhood distressing experiences, such as an intestinal disorder that was associated with fears of death.

In the last phase, we reprocessed the persisting triggers and her fears about the future concerning the upcoming birth of her grandchild. In total, the PTSD symptoms disappeared completely; at the time of her release, there remained only some mild depressive symptoms.

In a follow-up 6 months after her release, the patient showed no more depressive symptoms. She reported feeling very stable and was capable of handling trigger situations well. She reported having the feeling that, out of all the treatments she had experienced over the course of her life, inpatient EMDR therapy stabilized her the most and lasted over time.

This case and the one that follows are excellent examples of the problems that arise when there is a persisting comorbid trauma and a stress-related disorder that, if not recognized early on, subsequently leads to a more complicated treatment. In the following case, this also led to the patient's early retirement.

Case Study 8.2

TREATING A SPECIAL EDUCATION TEACHER WITH COMORBID TRAUMA AND DEPRESSIVE EPISODES WITH EMDR THERAPY

A 57-year-old special education teacher had depressive episodes as early as puberty, but only received the diagnosis of depression at age 34. She grew up in a household with many children. Her father was very strict to the point of violence and she was constantly anxious and had many nightmares. At 10 years old, she developed an eating disorder (anorexia) and was hospitalized for several months. During this time, she was isolated and for weeks contact with her family was prohibited.

After her diagnosis of depression, she had multiple outpatient, inpatient, and pharmaceutical treatment attempts that led only temporarily to an improvement. At 40, she retired early, and it was also in this context that she first received the diagnosis of PTSD; however, she only received trauma-specific treatment 10 years later from an outpatient psychotherapist who sent the patient to the hospital after a few months. During intake, the patient reported that she has had the feeling of "not being right" frequently, also of "not being right" in her body for a long time. She reported suffering from thoughts of inferiority, including self-hatred, and had issues of self-esteem. Often, she reported these feelings as overwhelming, particularly when in contact with those who were close to her. She also noted that she was anxious about frequently regressing into child-like emotional states. She noted feeling guilty about the way she was and got stressed and overwhelmed frequently. In addition, she had frequent thoughts of suicide. At the time she presented for therapy, she had been living for several months with a man who was 5 years older and her presenting problem was the increasing interpersonal difficulties with him.

After initially stabilizing the patient and strengthening her resources, we worked on establishing a Symptom Event Map and then targeted her pathogenic memories from childhood with EMDR therapy. The main focus was on her internal belief systems that contributed to many negative belief statements resulting in a very strong, self-critical attitude. After reprocessing, she felt considerable relief and developed new, positive attitudes. Additionally, we processed a situation with her partner in which she felt a line was crossed, and she ended up recognizing that she had the right to keep her boundaries and to respect her own needs. After this, the patient felt markedly surer of herself, including when her partner was in close physical proximity to her.

During a 6-month follow-up phone call, she indicated that she was still feeling noticeably more stable than before treatment. Although her relationship with her partner remained adversarial and there were external stressors such as end-of-life care for her father-in-law, she withstood these stressors and was able to respect her own boundaries. She reported that she had the feeling that she has really accomplished something in the last 6 months.

DEPRESSION AND SEVERE DISSOCIATIVE DISORDERS

In this form of depression, first described by Vedat Şar as dissociative depression, there is a severe dissociative disorder resulting from trauma, alongside recurrent or chronic depression (Şar, 2015). In treating dissociative depression, one must consider both the form of depression (chronic, recurrent) and its triggers, to the extent that they can be identified, as well as the dissociative disorder and the associated Depressive States that are almost always present. In working with these patients, the treatment of the dissociative disorder is usually given priority and treating the depression frequently takes a backseat, particularly at the beginning. An example for the treatment of dissociative depression is described in the following case.

Case Study 8.3

TREATING AN ADULT FEMALE DIAGNOSED WITH RECURRENT DEPRESSIVE, COMPLEX POSTTRAUMATIC STRESS DISORDERS AND SEVERE DISSOCIATIVE DISORDERS WITH EMDR THERAPY

A 29-year-old woman entered inpatient treatment with the diagnosis of recurrent depressive disorder, presently a moderate episode, complex trauma-related disorder, severe dissociative disorder, obsessive thoughts, obsessive behaviors, and anorexia nervosa. It was her sixth hospital stay in 10 years; during this time, she had also been in outpatient psychotherapy. She suffered from many issues: intrusions with physical responses, somatic difficulties, dissociative episodes with depersonalization and derealization, following several years of continued sexual abuse by her stepfather starting in elementary school. The reason for her current hospital stay was the death of her grandmother, who was her most important attachment figure. Given the highly complex, multi-morbid symptoms and her background of chronic and severe violence beginning in childhood in her family environment, the therapeutic process, which, as expected, was repeatedly punctuated with crises in the first few months, had to be organized in extremely small steps. The decisive factor in this process was the step-by-step increasing integration of the internal system of parts. Core elements of the therapeutic process were: disorder-specific psychoeducation, making internal connections, internally learning her parts and creating an internal "map," building up and improving internal communication, working from this base, and focusing and practicing specific possibilities of stabilization tailored to dissociation. We also conducted clearly defined trauma processing, in line with the current stabilization, but only in the second half of the 6-month hospital stay. This also led to an improvement of the patient's depressive and dissociative symptoms. EMDR could not be used during this first stay to process distressing memories because her dissociation was not well controlled and there was no tolerance for stimulation.

The decisive factor in this patient's case was the diagnosis of a dissociative identity disorder, since further planning for treatment in trauma-processing psychotherapy could only begin from understanding the importance of addressing this disorder first. In our experience, patients of this kind generally require multiple hospital stays or courses of psychotherapy before their tendency to relapse into severe, depressive symptoms can be resolved.

A comorbid dissociative disorder is not always a severe structural dissociative disorder (dissociative identity disorder or, according to the World Health Organization's *International Classification of Diseases*, 11th Edition [ICD-11], a partial dissociative identity disorder). There are also cases in which dissociative amnesia, without a deeper structural disorder, can be the cause for complications in treating a severe depressive episode. The following case is an example.

Case Study 8.4

TREATING A MOTHER WITH A LESS SEVERE DISSOCIATIVE DISORDER WITH EMDR THERAPY

A young mother of about age 30 was admitted to a psychiatric ward with a severe depressive episode and acute suicidality. It was the third and most severe depressive episode in 3 years. Therapeutic attempts remained without success for several weeks. The main problem was her chronic suicidality, that could barely be controlled even with an agreement to not engage in suicidal behaviors. The doctors spoke with the patient during their ward rounds and made a no-suicide agreement. Before the end of their round, they saw the patient, somewhat dazed, leave her room in an attempt to leave the ward with a clear suicidal intention. With no idea of what to do, the colleagues in the ward turned to an EMDR therapist in the hospital and asked him if he could perhaps help.

During history taking, there were no traumatic memories and no indications of a dissociative disorder. Somewhat helplessly, the therapist and patient searched for other distressing memories that could be a focus for EMDR. There were indications of moderately distressing memories of an orthopedic intervention during her youth. Since there was no other starting point, they focused on this memory and began the attempt to process the memory with EMDR. The distress at the beginning had a Subjective Units of Disturbance (SUD) of 5–6. After two sets of eye movements, a previously unremembered memory from childhood unexpectedly appeared. The patient remembered (again) for the first time a sexual assault by her father at age 5 that, up until that point, the patient had not remembered. In spite of the distress caused by processing the memory, the patient experienced noticeable relief already after the first session. Over the course of 15 additional EMDR therapy sessions, her suicidality and depression reduced considerably and disappeared entirely at the time of her discharge. Due to her remaining symptoms of trauma, she received outpatient, trauma-centered psychotherapy in the following years, also using EMDR. Due to a noticeably weaker depressive episode, she received inpatient EMDR therapy, once during this time, in which further childhood traumas and sexual assaults were processed with EMDR.

In a conversation over 20 years after the end of her first EMDR therapy, the patient reported that she was doing much better. She was capable of full-time work for 10 years and had not experienced any depressive episodes since. About her therapy, she said, "It is a long path, but it can be dealt with."

Overall, when treating depression, particularly those cases that do not respond to treatment, it is important to think about trauma-related disorders and dissociative disorders and to conduct appropriate diagnostics. The earlier an appropriate diagnosis is made for these patients, the more effective the following treatment can be. In the last case we described, which certainly represents an exception, an early, trauma-specific diagnosis would not have been very successful since the patient had complete amnesia of the childhood violence she experienced at that time. One would hope that a biological test to detect trauma and distress could be developed, precisely for making diagnoses in such cases. In the majority of cases, particularly in those of recurring and chronic depression, a simple diagnosis is sufficient to determine a comorbidity of trauma- and stressor-related disorders and to draw corresponding therapeutic conclusions.

In light of the fact that these patients not only suffer greatly from long hospital stays and year-long treatments, but also cause considerable problems for the healthcare system and are very expensive, there are perhaps in the medium-term institutions, e.g., insurers, who could further investigate this group of patients and the trauma-specific interventions that are necessary for them and integrate the results into the system of care.

REFERENCES

Anda, R. F., Felitti, V. J., Bremner, J. D., Walker, J. D., Whitfield, C. L., Perry, B. D., Dube, S. R., & Giles, W. H. (2006). The enduring effects of abuse and related adverse experiences in childhood: A convergence of evidence from neurobiology and epidemiology. *European Archives of Psychiatry and Clinical Neuroscience, 256*(3), 174–186. https://doi.org/10.1007/s00406-005-0624-4

Chen, L. P., Murad, M. H., Paras, M. L., Colbenson, K. M., Sattler, A. L., Goranson, E. N., Elamin, M. B., Seime, R. J., Shinozaki, G., Prokop, L. J., & Zirakzadeh, A. (2010). Sexual abuse and lifetime diagnosis of psychiatric disorders: Systematic review and meta-analysis. *Mayo Clinic Proceedings, 85*(7), 618–629. https://doi.org/10.4065/mcp.2009.0583

Cloitre, M., Hyland, P., Bisson, J. I., Brewin, C. R., Roberts, N. P., Karatzias, T., & Shevlin, M. (2019). ICD-11 posttraumatic stress disorder and complex posttraumatic stress disorder in the United States: A population-based study. *Journal of Traumatic Stress, 32*(6), 833–842. https://doi.org/10.1002/jts.22454

Gilbert, R., Widom, C. S., Browne, K., Fergusson, D., Webb, E., & Janson, S. (2009). Burden and consequences of child maltreatment in high-income countries. *The Lancet, 373*(9657), 68–81. https://doi.org/10.1016/S0140-6736(08)61706-7

Heim, C., Plotsky, P. M., & Nemeroff, C. B. (2004). Importance of studying the contributions of early adverse experience to neurobiological findings in depression. *Neuropsychopharmacology, 29*, 641–648. https://doi.org/10.1038/sj.npp.1300397

Jumper, S. A. (1995). A meta-analysis of the relationship of child sexual abuse to adult psychological adjustment. *Child Abuse & Neglect, 19*(6), 715–728. https://doi.org/10.1016/0145-2134(95)00029-8

Priebe, K., Kleindienst, N., Schropp, A., Dyer, A., Krüger-Gottschalk, A., Schmahl, C., Steil, R., & Bohus, M. (2019). Defining the index trauma in post-traumatic stress disorder patients with multiple trauma exposure: Impact on severity scores and treatment effects of using worst single incident versus multiple traumatic events. *European Journal of Psychotraumatology, 9*(1), Article 1486124. https://doi.org/10.1080/20008198.2018.1486124

Şar, V. (2015). Dissociative depression is resistant to treatment-as-usual. *Journal of Psychology & Clinical Psychiatry, 3*(2), Article 00128. https://doi.org/10.15406/jpcpy.2015.03.00128

Witt, A., Brown, R., Plener, P. L., Brähler, E., Fegert, J. M., & Clemens, V. (2019). Kindesmisshandlung und deren Langzeitfolgen: Analyse einer repräsentativen deutschen Stichprobe. *Zeitschrift für Psychiatrie, Psychologie und Psychotherapie, 67*(2), 100–111. https://doi.org/10.1024/1661-4747/a000378

Witt, A., Sachser, C., Plener, P. L., Brähler, E., & Fegert, J. M. (2019). The prevalence and consequences of adverse childhood experiences in the German population. *Deutsches Ärzteblatt, 116*, 635–642. https://doi.org/10.3238/arztebl.2019.0635

9

The EMDR-Drawing Integration (EMDR-DI) Protocol: A Visual Approach to Complex Posttraumatic Stress Disorder, Dissociation, and Depressive States

Gabriella Bertino, Luca Ostacoli, Sara Carletto, and Francesca Malandrone

INTRODUCTION

For the treatment of patients with complex depressive disorders with comorbidities and often significant psychosomatic symptoms, additional treatment tools are often very helpful.

Drawing is a useful way to represent trauma, supporting the differentiation between the adaptive and traumatized selves as a way to limit avoidance and dissociative reactions. It was first used to assist patients who were blocked in their ability to access traumatic material and who move between shut down and emotional arousal. Drawing was a less threatening way to first establish a sense of safety through body-based resources and then to enter the uncomfortable world of their traumatic experience. With the drawing as the image for the eye movement desensitization and reprocessing (EMDR) Assessment Phase, the rest of the assessment is accessed in the usual manner. Whenever a drawing is used, the Standard EMDR Protocol should be used later to be sure the material is fully reprocessed. The EMDR-Drawing Integration (EMDR-DI) Protocol is described, including case studies and patients' drawings.

THE EMDR-DRAWING INTEGRATION PROTOCOL

As a complement to the strategies already used in EMDR, drawing gives form to the inner representations of the trauma, objectifying it. In this way, people relate to something they can see, share, and concretely modify. Through the act of drawing, patients begin to differentiate between the adaptive ego and their traumatized emotional part. People may rapidly access preverbal and motor-sensory language, activating inborn creative skills. The use of such skills enables patients to access the traumatic material carefully, limiting dissociative reactions, bypassing avoidance and flight behaviors, and keeping a safe distance from the pain by objectifying it. The present chapter presents the EMDR-DI Protocol for use with various psychopathological conditions, such as dissociation, complex posttraumatic stress disorder (C-PTSD), and Depressive States, where it can help promote adaptive information processing in an effective manner.

This protocol is the product of several years of research and experimental applications of interventions using drawing integrated with EMDR. Initially, drawing was used by Ignacio Jarero and his team in Mexico where they drew on the ground with sticks while using what later became the EMDR Integrative Group Treatment Protocol (IGTP; Jarero et al., 1999). The use of drawing for the EMDR-DI was first employed as a "first aid" intervention in situations in which the management of responses to traumatic depression was difficult and often blocked by patients' defense reactions and their difficulty in accessing the traumatic material. Possible causes for this include the following:

- Traumatic material and the related emotions are frozen in a given time and space.
- Activated emotions, such as fear, sadness, anguish, grief, and anger, are at times overwhelming and persecutory, making them difficult for patients to manage.
- Traumatic material may cause patients to act in a threatening manner in the therapeutic relationship, endangering the therapeutic alliance.
- Dissociative reactions may result.

The initial goal of the integrated EMDR-DI was to allow patients to establish a sense of safety and stability, so that they could enter the destabilizing world of the traumatic experience while remaining connected. Any of these defense mechanisms can be activated by the instinctive need to feel safe and protected from something that feels too *painful or distressing*.

A sense of threat to subjects' integrity, that may be felt in the outside world (e.g., in their family or work relationships) and/or within their inner world (feelings, emotions), might lead them to say, "*It's too painful, I can't do it,*" or "*I'm afraid I won't be able to take it.*" Patients' requests, explicit or implicit, are that they need a protective boundary between the trauma and its associated emotions and their own self in order to be able to *see* and *hear* what is present from a position of safety. The patients' protective *boundary* is often the result of a tendency to ignore old feelings, not relive old memories, or the adoption of other strategies that permit subjects to avoid looking into their traumatic experience too deeply. It could also result from their feeling used to their pathological behaviors.

Sometimes individuals can no longer ignore the trauma, that the memories and emotions cannot continue to be held in a frozen state, or that defensive boundaries can no longer be maintained. When individuals open their *file* on the traumatic memory, they may become overwhelmed, unable to give shape, substance, or color to their illness, and often present with a set of generalized symptoms. In an attempt to defend themselves, people may try to cling to a rigid set of negative beliefs concerning their relationship with themselves, with others, or

Chapter 9   The EMDR-Drawing Integration (EMDR-DI) Protocol   147

with the world in general, in order to establish a sense of security—even if it is only present on a cognitive level. Alternatively, they may find themselves remaining entangled in relationships characterized by suffering and abuse.

Entering into the internal space of the trauma involves the risk of losing the real and healthy boundaries of the self, with the clear danger of being totally absorbed by the trauma, as if a black hole were present that attracts, traps, and envelops the self in a dimension of total loneliness.

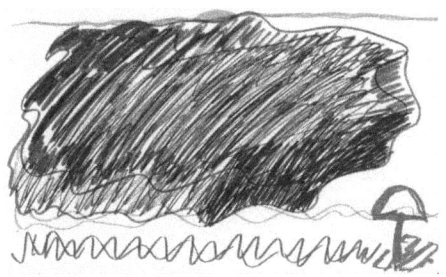

FIGURE 9.1 Drawing by adult female patient depicts the fear of her trauma.

In Figure 9.1, an adult female patient draws the fear of her trauma and says, *"Anguish is like a black stain that covers everything and crushes me. I have no means of escape. Freezing is the only way to protect myself from fear and pain ... I am frozen and protected, the waves lull me ... But can I even exist and be alive? ..."*

Here, by representing herself and her defense mechanisms, the patient can build a bridge between the *I can't exist* and the *I want to exist*. How does the approach with drawing help overcome these situations of deadlock and circumvent the defense mechanisms without putting the person in a state of danger? How is drawing able to activate strong security boundaries and adaptive skills that allow for processing and integration?

WHAT HAPPENS DURING THE ACT OF DRAWING?

Drawing helps subjects to give shape, color, and movement to their internal representation of the trauma by allowing them to relate to the traumatic material as something real that can be seen, represented, and touched. It helps create a solid protective boundary between the self (that must stabilize, strengthen, and consolidate itself) and that piece of their history (that needs to be dealt with) but parts of the self are blocked.

In the act of drawing, patients make an initial symbolic representation and reorganization of the shape of the trauma, and then they can start to distinguish their adaptive self that has the tools and the ability to restructure the experiences, while their traumatic emotional part remains in a state of helplessness and passivity. The process is made possible by accessing pre-verbal and sensorimotor language, that activates the innate creative abilities (Fisher, 2017). They no longer feel overwhelmed by the traumatic experience, made up of memories, images, emotions and feelings, and they can activate their adaptive capacities because they are enveloped by the sensation of being in a state of complete safety.

The act of drawing the traumatic experience and the actual drawing in its final representation becomes an important link between the perception of patients' inner reality—their emotions, feelings, beliefs, images, and so on—and their external reality, where they now have the possibility to freely share the experience with another person. Thus, drawing allows subjects to explore and describe their inner material, giving it form and color within its own objective space. The value of the drawing is not in its *aesthetics*, but in its capacity to enhance internal processing by means of the graphic gestures made that create a representation of the memory and the traumatic experience. Sometimes even very minimalistic drawings composed of simple signs (lines, circles, or spots) can be enough to generate rich inner elaboration, because the graphics originate from and are connected to an internal urge, a desire to give shape and color to something that is often undefined and undifferentiated.

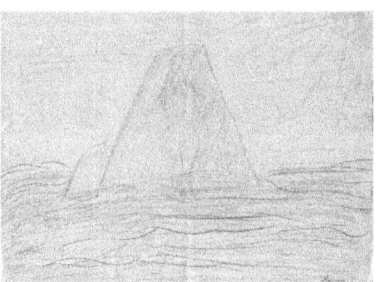

FIGURE 9.2 Freezing: An adult female patient draws how the defense of freezing protects her.

In Figure 9.2, an adult patient draws how freezing protects her: *"Freezing becomes the only way to protect myself from pain and fear. ... I'm frozen and protected, the sea waves lull me ... but can I exist and be alive?..."* In this case, by representing herself and her defense mechanism, the subject can build a bridge between *"I can't exist"* and *"I want to exist."* In this particular subject, the work with EMDR continued, focusing on her defense mechanism

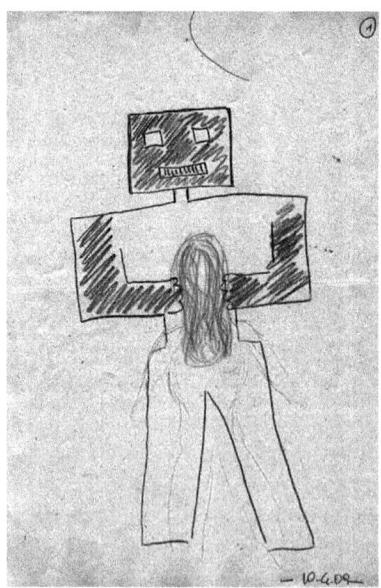

FIGURE 9.3 An adult patient depicts how she is a prisoner in her head.

In Figure 9.3, an adult patient depicts how she is a prisoner in her head: *"My head is locked. I am a prisoner of my thoughts, my fears. As if some outside force is holding me down. Where am I? ... I exist only in my head."* By means of this representation, it becomes possible for the person to confront the power of the rational part that controls, directs, and blocks the vitality experience. She now focuses her attention on making her body, its forms and its needs, the object. Drawing has allowed her to initiate a dialogue of the different sides, and through working with EMDR she can now begin to address linked episodes, representing blocking beliefs and bringing about change.

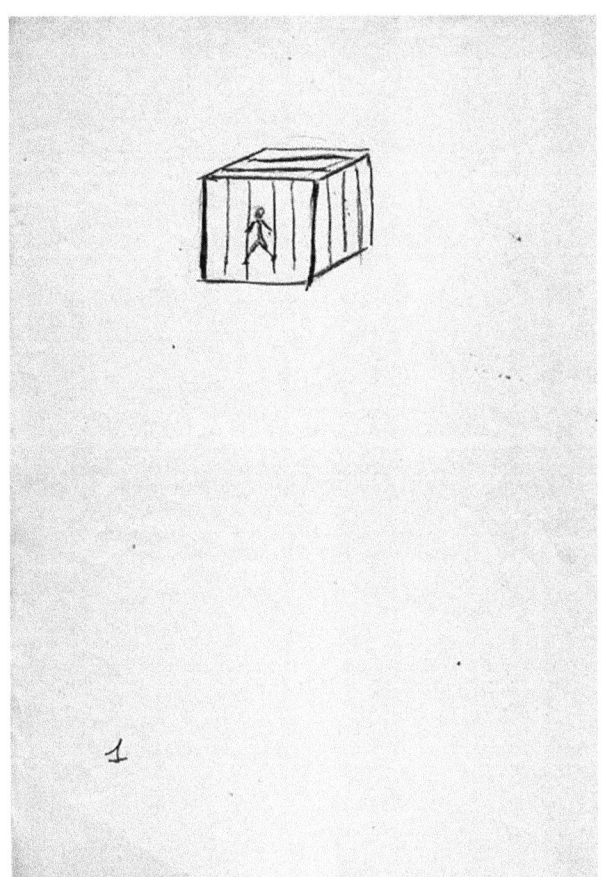

FIGURE 9.4 A severely depressed man draws how *locked* he feels.

In Figure 9.4, a severely depressed man draws how *locked* he feels. This drawing portrays the *locked* condition in a man with severe depression. However, the act of drawing this representation has sparked the patient's desire to change. *"It's a moment of great crisis and of blockage, a sense of failure, and lack of physical and mental energy and inability to react. I'm trapped inside a cage, closed in. Someone has put a weight on my shoulders, a stone that weighs me down. I'm inadequate."*

A short example of a potential therapeutic dialogue:

Therapist: *Where would you like to see yourself?*
Patient: *Out of the cage, I'd love to see him in a boat ... in a boat rowing, so that he can move forward and overcome the difficulties formed by the waves and the wind ...*
Therapist: *Try to draw it.*
The patient draws.
Patient: *When I concentrate on this drawing, I notice how I stiffen.*
The patient uses the method of tapping and the tension eases.
Patient: *Something is stabilizing inside me right now.*

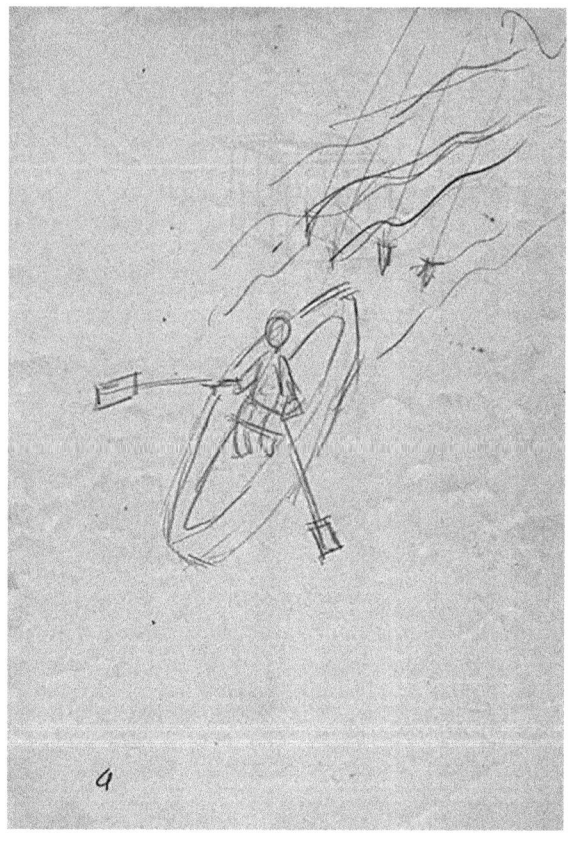

FIGURE 9.5 A male patient uses his dream to inspire a drawing to help him move forward.

In Figure 9.5, a male patient uses his dream to inspire a drawing to help him move forward. The change that the patient dreams of, speculated, and then verbalized thanks to the drawing, takes form. It becomes an adaptive part of the self, occupying a space that is initially physical and then mental. The drawing of the image and the stimulation has set a self-healing process in motion.

THE TECHNIQUE: EMDR-DRAWING INTEGRATION PROTOCOL

Here are the steps of the EMDR-DI Protocol:

- Definition of the target (the worst episode or, in some cases, the present moment experience) and definition of the worst image (treated as the image of the Standard EMDR Protocol).
- Clinicians tells the clients: *"Visualize your worse image and draw it."*
- Therapists provide clients with a large sheet of paper, felt-tip pens, colored pencils, and crayons.

  Note: The variety of drawing materials is crucial because the process is different depending on the material used. Felt-tip pens make decisive lines, providing greater impact; colored pencils allow the client to represent the image very delicately, sometimes the drawing is almost imperceptible, limiting the drawing's impact. Crayons allow clients to apply strength and give the image motion, permitting a greater breadth of expression and the intermingling of colors.

- It is important that at the end of each drawing, people put all the colors they used back in order, so that they feel free to choose from the whole range of materials and colors for the next drawing.
- If clients are hesitating too much, therapists could help them by saying, *"Don't worry, let your hand choose the color and just let it express on the sheet what is happening inside you right now, as freely as you can. You don't need to know how to draw, it doesn't need to be aesthetically pleasing, just let the worst image that exists within you take form on the paper, using the colors that come to you instinctively."*
- You can support the process by saying: *"You're doing well."*
- Complete the assessment of the drawn image and include the negative cognition, positive cognition, Validity of Cognition (VOC), Emotion, Subjective Units of Disturbance (SUD), and Body Location.
- Clinicians ask clients to focus on the drawing, on the negative cognition and on where within their body they sense that the emotions are localized while performing bilateral stimulation.
- At the end of each set, the completed drawing or the drawing in progress is briefly investigated by asking clients questions, such as, *"What do you notice? What do you feel? What does that say about you? What is going on inside you now,"* and so on. The subject then proceeds with new drawings. If the questions prompt a change in the clients, they may modify the drawing or, if the change is radical, clients may want to represent it in a new drawing.
- After several sets and drawings, an adaptive representation usually emerges that can be installed as a resource.
- In subsequent sessions, therapists ask clients to return to the event: *"Recall the event and note what is happening within you now ... try to draw it."*

It is important to underline that when a traumatic event with a crucial role in the history of the person has been processed through the integration of the drawing material, it is necessary at a later stage to resume the processing with the Standard EMDR Protocol, without the use of the drawing. For example, it is analogous to situations when clients were taking antidepressant drugs. After stopping the medication, it is important to reprocess the material. Both the drawing and the drug, in fact, may mask important emotions; therefore, there may be more emotions to process. Generally, when the event is re-accessed, the process is quick and allows for the resolution of the target. This is only necessary for targets with a central role in the person's history.

USING THE EMDR-DRAWING INTEGRATION PROTOCOL IN DIFFICULT SITUATIONS

It is possible to use the drawing tool within a desensitization/reprocessing session when blocking conditions, deadlocks, dissociation, or overwhelming emotions present themselves in the following way:

- Clinicians invite clients to focus on what is happening in the *here and now*. If clients are in trouble, therapists could support them by saying, "*Don't worry, let your hand choose the right color and let it start drawing what is happening inside you right now, the goal is not to make a beautiful drawing, you don't need to know how to draw, just let whatever wants to come out do so.*"
- Therapists can support the process by stating, "*You are doing well.*"
- Once clients have finished drawing, therapists ask them to comment on it. They should be allowed to describe what they have drawn, but not attempt to interpret it (the idea is to treat the graphical representation as the material that emerges during the process of desensitization).
- Key questions to ask about the drawing and about what took place during the drawing process:
    - "*What do you notice?*"
    - "*What do you feel?*"
    - "*What is happening inside you now?*"
    - "*What does it say about you?*"
- Clients are then asked to focus on the drawing and therapists work with eye movements or with tapping.
- If clients experience strong activation while drawing, support the drawing process with soft tapping on their knees (with advance permission) or shoulders—like a hug that supports and contains. In general, it is better to distinguish the two moments and leave clients their own personal space to complete the drawing and then therapists may intervene with a set of bilateral stimulation.

In summary, the use of drawing with respect to trauma allows us to:

- Create objective conditions for safety to access the traumatic material in a *protected* manner.
- Shape and objectify the traumatic material in a sharing relationship with therapists.
- Create a space of protection between the self and the part that is the bearer of suffering.
- Access, in a protected way, the traumatic material avoiding the activation of dissociative behaviors.

Chapter 9 The EMDR-Drawing Integration (EMDR-DI) Protocol

- Give voice and power to the inner child, accessing the first forms of child-like communication.
- See how reprocessing is illustrated concretely through drawings and shows a change of perception in patients.
- Install resources both as adaptive images and as confidence in one's own creative abilities.
- Reduce any destabilization following incomplete sessions by focusing on the drawing of the trauma instead of the inner image of the trauma; this reduces the emotional activation.

> **Box 9.1.** The EMDR-Drawing Integration Protocol: A Testimony About a Patient's Journey Through the Horrors of Childhood With the Aid of Drawing
>
> *Drawing helped me to make contact with my traumatic memory, and to transform the fear, the terror, and the sense of annihilation into a color that could then fade, into an outline that defines a form that represents the horror and the destruction of the child self, suffocated by the weight of the monstrous form that hides the love, left to a world without hope.*
>
> *The lines and the colors are like anchors, letting me stay in touch with the here and now, with the healthy parts of myself. Like oars rowing in the right direction, like the dot on a map that tells you where you are and shows you the way to go (...). It's like being inside a protective shell that allows you to make contact with harmful substances, while keeping the healthy parts safe (...). For me, drawing was like having a companion, a spiritual guide who followed me into the cave of my horrors, whispering to me, "You can learn to protect yourself."*

EXPLORING THE DEPRESSIVE STATES WITH THE EMDR-DRAWING INTEGRATION PROTOCOL

In our view, there are essentially two types of Depressive States:

- *Cold States:* Entirely *cold*, characterized by apathy, insensitivity, ideomotor slowdown; some patients describe themselves as being *potatoes* without any emotion. They are typical of the bipolar spectrum. When these disorders occur in acute form, the psychotherapeutic possibilities are very limited, the reprocessing of life events is postponed during the crisis, and patients' psychological goals aim at supporting daily routines, while maintaining connections with important family members.
- *Mixed States: Mixed* between aspects of shut down and emotional arousal; when emotions appear they are generally about loss of meaning or melancholy. The EMDR-DI is most helpful with this state.

Depressive States represent highly uncomfortable experiences. People feel completely overwhelmed, and if there are moments of serenity, they are not remembered or they are experienced as something ephemeral without consistency. From the temporal perspective, patients feel that they have always felt like this and they will always be like this. From the spatial vantage, patients feel lost in a dimension of suffering that is very vast and detached from the reality of others, so that help is perceived as fundamentally useless. The emotional experience is one of desperation, without seeing any way out. Depressive States represent a paradox because despite this dimension of suffering that distances people from everything and everyone, especially from themselves, they are often perceived at the same time as something very familiar that has always accompanied that person, with a profound intimacy.

The procedure we propose is three steps: focus on the incident, exploration, and acceptance of one's experience to a greater extent than in the Standard EMDR Assessment. The Depressive State is a recurring state that the person has been in and will be in many times more. *The main objective is not to change the state at once, but first look at it in "relationship" with the worst state that clients experience.*

PREPARATORY ASSESSMENT: THE SELF-CONTACT TECHNIQUE

Before processing memories, an assessment about stability has to be made. The preparatory assessment is based on the assessment through the Self-Contact Technique described in Chapter 3 and in the following. There are three stages of stability or instability which use traffic light colors to signal if the processing of memories can start, continue, or stop.

1. *Green Light:* People feel grounded, with at least one of their two hands in contact with the body, without discomfort. The three described phases of Representation, Staying in Contact and Acceptance, and Elaboration, can be followed when there is a green light.
2. *Yellow Light:* People can experience being grounded and at least one of their two hands is in contact with the body without discomfort, after stabilization practices such as grounding or others. In this case, the second phase of Staying in Contact and Acceptance must be done by carefully monitoring the state of arousal and, if they tend to go out of the window of tolerance, they bring it back inside. This is the meaning of the yellow light.
3. *Red Light:* These people are not grounded and/or the contact of both hands is perceived with discomfort or they do not feel the contact: There is a high probability that they are in a dissociative state. In this case, the phases of Representation and Elaboration can be carried out but not the one of Staying in Contact and Acceptance; this will be postponed until people will have recovered a sense of physical boundaries and some capacity to feel empathy toward themselves.

The practice of exploring and accepting the Depressive State helps to expand resilience: The more that is learned about the state, the more possible it is to accept it, and the less people will be conditioned to react maladaptively to it. The more people fight against it, the more they are stuck. *It is important not to try to get results,* but *sit with yourself,* notice and accept what happens, as if you were sitting in the cinema and looking at the screen, or on a train and watching the landscape go by the window, or on the bank of a river watching the water flow. It is not a relaxation technique. It is a moment of encounter with yourself, where, if you accept your emotions, it will bring you partial relief. Think about your worst emotional experience in just the way it is, without looking for anything special, just accepting whatever happens or does not happen, it is fine just the way it is.

Chapter 9 The EMDR-Drawing Integration (EMDR-DI) Protocol

In our protocol we approach Depressive States with a three-step procedure:

- Representation
- Exploration With an Attitude of Acceptance
- Processing

1. Representation
Representation includes observation and representation. The first step is *not* to try to modify Depressive States but rather to represent them, by exploring their qualities and being an observer. In this way, patients can step back and instead of *being encompassed* by these states they can *enter into a relationship* with their own worst experience. Patients subjected to Depressive States feel these states many times; therefore, it is essential to familiarize and reduce their reactivity by increasing the sense of control before entering the second step: processing with an accepting attitude. Exploring the Depressive State together also brings them back into the relationship.

The Self-Contact Technique: The technique is similar to Katie O'Shea's protocol (Paulsen et al., 2017) to prepare patients to regulate their emotions. For this, explore the Depressive State, starting either from the image or the emotional experience of the state to then studying the other elements of the experience, emphasizing those to which patients find the easiest to respond, such as the following:

- If the state was represented by an image, what would it be?
- If the state had a shape, color, and/or sound, what would it be?
- Invite patients to represent the image on a sheet of paper, according to the EMDR-DI described previously. The representation sometimes is very detailed, while others are very simple, even just a few lines or a color.
- Check patients' connection between the representation and their own experience.
- Patients put their hands at the sides of the drawing sheet and look at the image.
- The therapist does four to six sets of tapping.
- After each set, ask if there is something that they could add or change so that the image would better represent their experience.

Note: Usually at the beginning, patients modify the image.

- Therapists repeat the process until the representation remains unchanged for at least two successive sets. The tapping must be very short to avoid triggering the reprocessing. The goal is not to reduce discomfort but to become aware of the characteristics of the emotional state; as a result, a SUD is not taken.

2. Exploration With an Attitude of Acceptance
Once the experience has been represented and it has been verified that it corresponds to the experience of the Depressive State, it is very important to help people explore it with an accepting attitude. In this way, the reactivity to the emotional state is reduced and self-efficacy is strengthened. There is a more realistic understanding that the fight–flight behavior is not helpful, and learning to live with it without too much fear occurs. Again, it is also important in this step not to try to change the state, otherwise patients enter a fight–flight relationship that blocks the process.

Note: It is surprising how many times the discomfort is reduced when patients no longer fight against the state and take the stance of an accepting observer. The accepting attitude was founded in approaches based on Mindfulness and Compassion; these approaches are helpful in reducing symptoms in a way comparable to psychotherapy in mild and moderate forms of depression and are an important part of the EMDR approach to depression. Many of the blocks in therapy occur precisely because the therapist tries to *change* the people's experience, instead of encountering it together and accepting it as it is, and helping patients to stay in the encounter by adjusting the arousal level so that it remains within the window of tolerance. Krupnik (2018) developed a protocol that uses a similar principle that he called Treating Depression Downhill (TDD).

Once there is a representative image for the Depressive State and it corresponds to peoples' experiences, it is very important to help them explore and welcome it. Since it is a predominantly emotional, bodily experience, it is often useful to explore it from the bottom-up sequence, from physical sensations then emotion(s) then thought(s).

> **Box 9.2.** The EMDR-Drawing Integration Protocol: Script to Explore a Patient's Depressive State With an Attitude of Acceptance

1. Open awareness to the represented Depressive State.
Therapist: *Choose if you want to close your eyes or keep them open and while you are looking at the image that represents the emotional state that creates the most difficulty for you, try to recall the experience and, if you would like, explore it with curiosity, feeling all the support and caring that is possible in this moment toward yourself.*

2. Explore physical sensations.
Tapping:
Therapist: *By closing your eyes, notice where you feel the most discomfort—your abdomen, your chest, your stomach, your throat—then you can gently explore what the physical sensation is like—for example, does it feel oppressive, tense, empty, contracted, or something else? If you have the impression of feeling nothing/numb, be aware of that, and allow yourself to feel what you feel or the lack of feeling.*

Now, you can open your eyes; What do you notice?

Stay with that.
Use bilateral stimulation.

3. Notice emotional tone.
Tapping:
Therapist: *Now, notice the emotions you are feeling. Is it closer to fear, to frustration, anger, or sadness—or perhaps you are numb. Simply notice what is in this moment, just as it is.*

Now, you can open your eyes again. What do you notice?
Stay with that.
Use bilateral stimulation.

4. Explore thoughts.
As you think about the image ask:
Therapist: *What's the worst part about it? Listen as the question slowly reverberates in your mind, and take some breaths while you go with that.*
Do bilateral stimulation.
What do you notice?
Stay with that.
Do bilateral stimulation.

5. Accepting the experience of the Depressive State like the sky and the clouds that pass by.
Tapping:
Therapist: *At this important moment, maybe the most important of all, notice what emotions or numbness you are experiencing and, if you like, you can experience them as messages that really come from yourself, to help you, and you can welcome the experience you are having, whatever it may be.*

Remember that you are greater that any emotion you can feel—the feelings of discomfort are clouds that pass by—you can be the sky that accepts and welcomes everything—sun and rain are part of life—and even if everything becomes dark sometimes and there is wind and thunder—it is just a storm—and by remembering you are the sky—much greater than any cloud that may pass by—you can accept what is happening—gently—breathing and feeling inside the abdomen that fills by inhaling—and you can welcome the experience you are having, whatever it may be, telling it, "I feel you, take all the space you need for as long as you like, you are welcome." You can let the welcome resonate slowly 5 or 6 times, with at least two breaths between each one: "I feel you, take all the space you need for as long as you like, you are welcome."

What do you notice?
Stay with that.
Do bilateral stimulation.

The tapping and the welcoming sentence can be repeated, if needed.
If the image has changed after acceptance work, you can ask patients to do a new drawing to represent their new experience.

3. Processing
After you have explored the Depressive State and strengthened the position of the accepting observer, proceed to the processing of the state itself, according to the EMDR-DI Protocol, as previously described.

Case Study 9.1

THE EMDR-DRAWING INTEGRATION PROTOCOL WHEN WORKING WITH DEPRESSIVE STATES

Symptoms and Emotional Experiences: *Luisa is a 22-year-old student working on her degree in social services. She presented with symptoms of depression and dissociation, such as getting stuck, feeling detached from the people around her, and experiencing that everything seems meaningless. She felt emotionally empty with moments of intense melancholy of which she did not know the meaning. She was afraid she would be swallowed up by these states.*

Anamnesis: *She was involved with a young man who showed behavior consistent with narcissistic, dominant, and often violent personality disorders: He often exposed Luisa to verbal, as well as physical, threats, if she did not follow exactly what he ordered her to do. Although she was afraid of his behavior, she could not leave him and this caused her great conflict with her family, who were affectionate, connected, and very worried about this relationship.*

Luisa could not detach herself from him because, as she stated, the time spent with him was the only time she felt she existed. It is in this sort of folie à deux where she alternated between intense feelings of love and fear of him that she felt truly alive, at least for a moment. All this was associated with a sort of moral duty that led her to try to save her boyfriend, as if he could not survive without her. Luisa found no peace in her life and even the people closest to her, her classmates and friends, were perceived as dull, lacking true vitality, in a normal world to which she felt she did not belong. She generally perceived her relationships in a detached way without any emotional participation, except for melancholy.

Assessment: *Red Light: When her feet were grounded and her hands felt connected to her body, she was uncomfortable. She felt lost in space and without any boundary that defined her body. This did not improve with grounding techniques; she actually tended to get worse.*

Processing Through EMDR Drawing Integration:

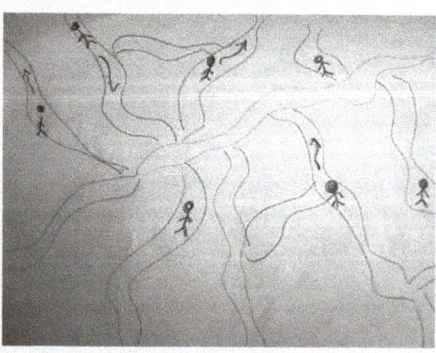

FIGURE 9.6 The graphic representation of a patient's emotional experience of being part of a meaningless world.

Chapter 9 The EMDR-Drawing Integration (EMDR-DI) Protocol

In Figure 9.6, the patient draws a representation of her being part of a meaningless world: The only exceptions were the extremely intense moments she experienced with her boyfriend; even though they were often dangerous, they were the only ones where she felt alive. Otherwise, her life was a space without boundaries, devoid of color, in which people moved like automatons moving away from each other, without direction.

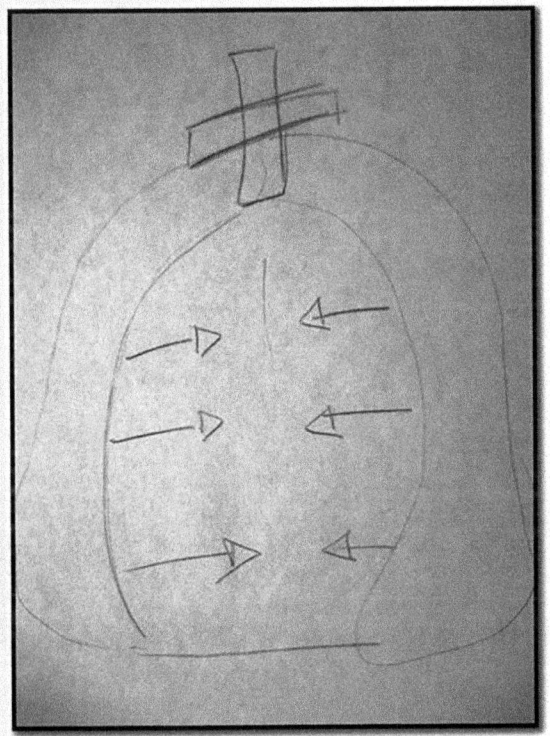

FIGURE 9.7 Luisa's depiction of her body as an empty shell.

In Figure 9.7, Luisa used her drawing to depict her representation of her body. **Luisa:** *It was just an empty shell.* (Initially, there were no arrows. The drawing gets more complete as the process continued.)

Therapist: *Go with that.*

Therapist used bilateral stimulation.

Then, she added the arrows. She perceived her body as she felt this pressure toward the inside: There was no boundary, there was no edge.

Therapist: *Go with that.*

Therapist used bilateral stimulation, after the drawing and description.

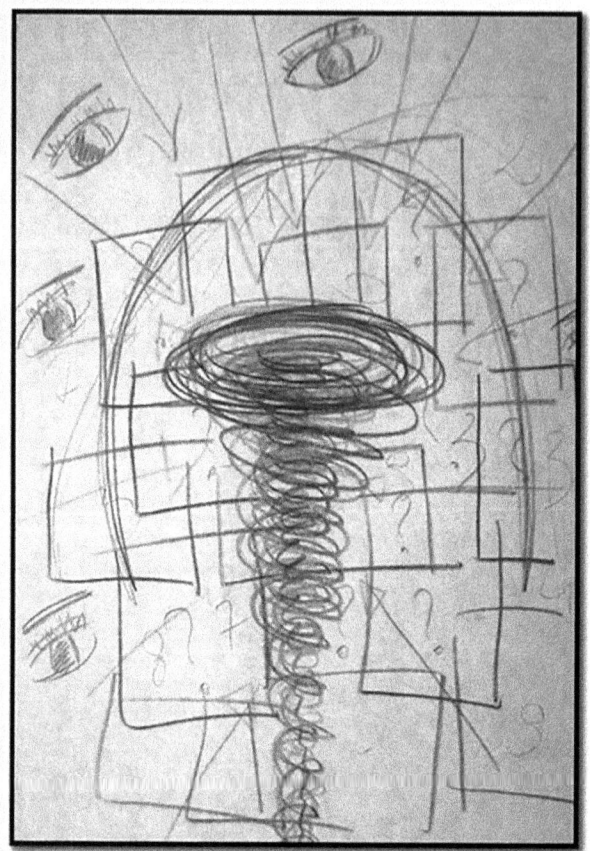

FIGURE 9.8 Luisa's changing representation of her body without and with boundaries.

In Figure 9.8, Luisa shows the evolution of her experience of boundaries concerning her own body. At first, there were no eyes or arrows or tornadoes. There were only unrelated geometric lines and random numbers. Initially, the drawing gets more complete in the process.

Luisa: *My body is without boundaries and absurd.*

Therapist used bilateral stimulation, after the drawing and description.

Then, Luisa added eyes and red arrows. The looks of people close to her were the only things she began to perceive as vague boundaries.
Therapist used bilateral stimulation, after the drawing and description.
Luisa added the tornado.

Luisa: *I feel this tornado threatening to absorb me like a black hole. I feel powerless.*

Therapist used bilateral stimulation, after the drawing and description.

Chapter 9 The EMDR-Drawing Integration (EMDR-DI) Protocol **161**

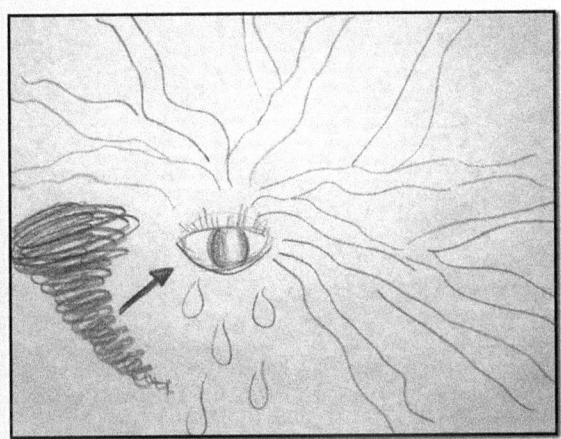

FIGURE 9.9 Luisa uses her drawing to show the evolution of feelings in herself.

In Figure 9.9, Luisa uses her drawing to show the evolution of feelings in herself. In the beginning, initially, there were no tears or a tornado. In this drawing, the initial image, Figure 9.5 with the different roads, seemed to be revisited. Now, the roads started from the eye in the center of the drawing.

Therapist used bilateral stimulation, after the drawing and description.
Luisa added tears. This time, however, all those roads were no longer meaningless, but a feeling began to appear of sadness represented by tears.

Therapist: *What is this sadness?*

Therapist used bilateral stimulation.
Luisa added the tornado.

Luisa: *It is the fear of getting lost in the tornado; it threatens me, but I can see it.*

Therapist used 2 or 3 sets of bilateral stimulation.

More and more emotion emerged.

In Figure 9.10, Luisa charts her ability to begin to connect with others. At first, there were neither blue lines nor drops, only houses and people.

Luisa: *All the people have a body, and a house while I have nothing.*

Therapist used bilateral stimulation.
Luisa drew the blue lines.

Luisa: *They are like the wind that passes through everything and leaves no trace.*

Therapist used bilateral stimulation.

Luisa: *The wind transforms, it becomes rain drops that come down.*

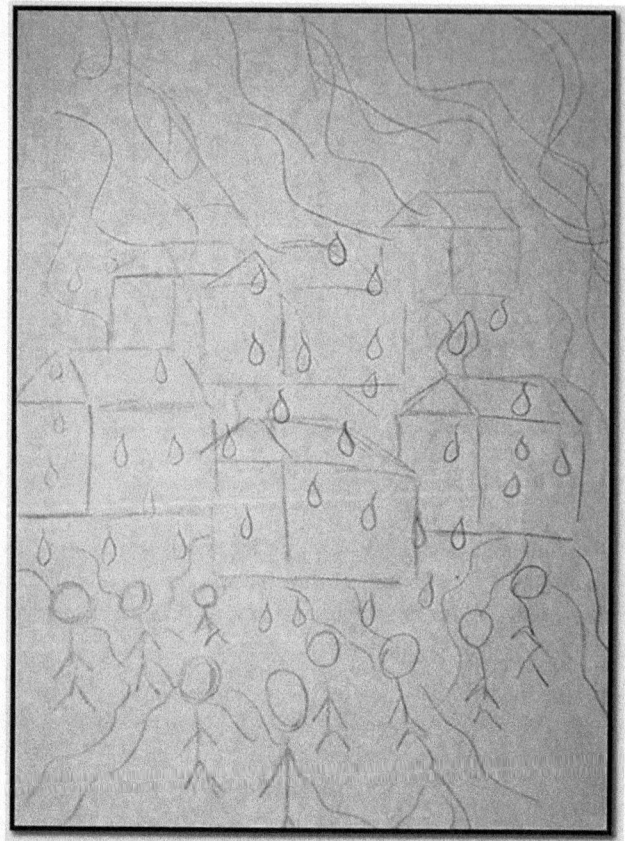

FIGURE 9.10 Luisa depicts her emerging ability to connect with others.

Therapist used bilateral stimulation.

Luisa: *These raindrops touch everything.*

Therapist used bilateral stimulation.

Luisa: *The drops melt when they touch things.*

While she said this, Luisa paused for a moment, and the therapist felt the emergence of a delicate emotion. It was the first time that she used a term that implied a contact. The therapist used the technique of focusing on the exact moment in which the drop touched what it encountered.

Therapist: *Pay attention to the moment when the drops touch everything and melt away.*

Therapist used bilateral stimulation.
Luisa underwent a transformation in her body, as did the expression in her face.

Chapter 9   The EMDR-Drawing Integration (EMDR-DI) Protocol

It tended to melt a bit, like the drops during contact then emotion emerged.
Therapist used bilateral stimulation.
For the first time, Luisa said, she felt peace inside.

Therapist used bilateral stimulation on the contact of the drops, their melting, and becoming one with what they touched, the sense of peace of this merging.
The feeling of peace and relaxation increased, like something Luisa had not felt for a long time.
Therapist used bilateral stimulation.
Therapist: *Try to stay with this feeling, let it flow throughout your body, experiencing it, in every single cell.*
Therapist used bilateral stimulation.

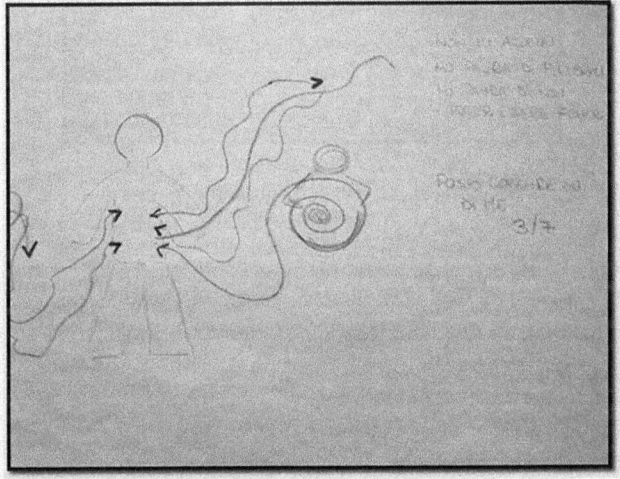

FIGURE 9.11 Luisa's drawing shows her difficulty accepting and counting on herself.

In Figure 9.11, Luisa draws her difficulty accepting and counting on herself. At first, there was no writing and no arrows. After that, a body took shape in the drawing: there were no feet, no hands, and no eyes. The face was empty, but later there were raindrops coming out of the face.

Therapist used bilateral stimulation.
Luisa added arrows facing inward.

Luisa: *I absorb everything like a sponge, everything enters me, I reverberate with everything.*
Therapist used bilateral stimulation.
Luisa: *I don't accept myself, I'm afraid of losing myself, I'm afraid of not being able to be happy.* A positive cognition with VOC of 3/7 appears: *I can count on myself.*

The boundaries of Luisa's body were not defined yet, there was no contact with the ground, she was sad; she seemed to have no protection from what resonated inside, and a great vulnerability started to emerge.
Therapist used bilateral stimulation.

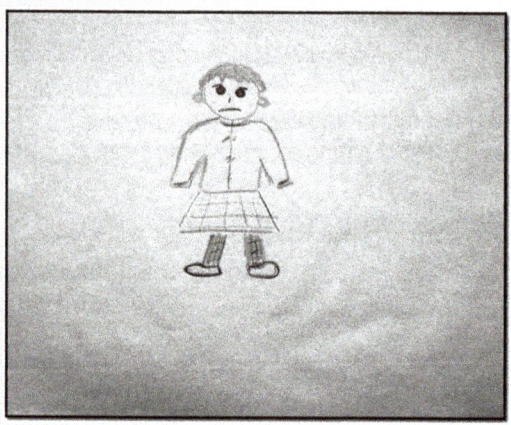

FIGURE 9.12 Luisa's emerging anger; feet planted on the ground emerge.

In Figure 9.12, Luisa begins to show her anger and emerging connection in the present.
Initially, her drawing was without feet. She started to feel a different emotion other than sadness; anger appeared.
Therapist used bilateral stimulation.
Luisa drew the feet and she drew anger on her face.
Therapist used bilateral stimulation.
Luisa drew the buttons on her shirt.
Therapist used bilateral stimulation.

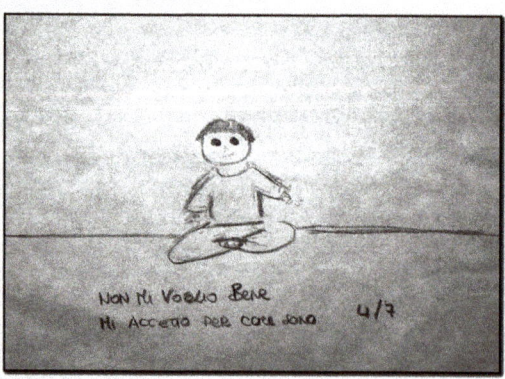

FIGURE 9.13. Luisa began to depict her ability to be in contact with the ground and her own body.

In Figure 9.13, Luisa shows in her body her growing ability to connect with the ground and her own body. Initially, there was no writing. This drawing went back to having just one color. There were feet and a light depiction of hands. She drew the ground and she had contact with the grounding position through her crossed legs.

Luisa: *I feel more stable.*
Therapist used bilateral stimulation.
Therapist: *What does this image say about you?*
Therapist used bilateral stimulation.
She added the writing, and then the cognitions.
Luisa: Negative cognition: *I don't love myself.* Positive cognition: *I accept myself as I am.* VOC equals 4/7.

Now, Luisa was able to feel the contact of the feet with the ground a bit and the touch of one of her two hands on her body.

Commentary:
By using the EMDR-DI Protocol, Luisa began to have a better sense of her spatial boundaries and internal representation of herself, allowing future work to proceed according to the Standard EMDR Protocol.

The drawings, in addition to supporting the exploration of disorders with a dissociative tendency, allowed us to view through her drawings the process of Luisa's stabilization. By the end, the hands and feet of the figure were no longer suspended, but she was sitting on a floor. With the recovery of body boundaries, cognitions began to emerge more clearly, and she was able to process what was going on with less need to use drawing as a stabilization aid. The therapy continued with the Standard EMDR Protocol.

After a few sessions, Luisa reported feeling physical pain in the form of a cold feeling on the left side of her chest. By focusing on the sensation, the cold increased. Using an affect bridge, she followed the pain and the cold feeling. Initially, there was only cold and pain, accompanied by a sense of alarm. Using short, light bilateral stimulations, and making sure she was grounded so she did not dissociate, she accessed a memory that she had been in an incubator for a period of 2 months when she was born. She had no images of this, but did know that it was an actual event that happened in her life. She felt that the pain she felt today was connected to what happened to her then. As she deepened the association, through bilateral stimulation, it emerged that the pain was a memory that came from an intravenous feeding tube, and the cold was from the absence of human contact.

Note: At the time Luisa was born, there was minimal touching of newborns in the incubator, due to fear of infections, so infants remained isolated in the incubators. The absence of bodily contact for prolonged periods of time impaired the infant's ability to develop a sense of her body's boundaries. These boundaries later would have helped support the infant's basic understanding of emotions. Today, we know that bodily contact with parents does not cause any negative effects. Touching improves the maturation of the nervous system and the recovery of the newborns. In most neonatal intensive care units, *kangaroo therapy* is practiced with skin-to-skin contact.

After this revelation, the therapist decided to use a guided visualization to support processing from both perspectives of the here and now and there and then:

Imagine you are next to the incubator and observe that the child is being fed intravenously in the left part of her chest. Nobody could touch her for fear of infections. Now, look at her with today's eyes from your adult self and become aware of what you feel toward the child, then as you identify with what the newborn feels, feel the coldness and how alone she felt.

The therapist then had her pendulate between the adult part and the baby part, while using tapping.

After a while, the therapist asked the adult part to imagine doing what was not done for her at the time and was what she needed. Louisa chose to touch and hold that baby. During the bilateral stimulation, Luisa began gradually to feel a tenderness that was accompanied by a feeling of relaxation in her body. Then, the therapist had her imagine picking up that younger child and placing her on her chest to welcome and protect her, accompanied by BLS.

Luisa began to feel a growing sense of union and well-being and the expression on her face and posture changed. She looked progressively more nurturing. When she imagined herself as the mother holding the baby, a sense of complete peace emerged. The negative cognition was transformed and became *I love you and I accept you as you are*, and the VOC became 6/7.

At this time, the therapist did the *Daily Life Experience Test*, which checks if patients are able to talk about their daily life stresses without decompensating (Hofmann, 2009). Luisa did much better now. She understood that the Depressive State was not an existential state but it was the call of little Luisa who needed to be accepted. If there were a re-emergence of the feeling of loss of meaning and deep loneliness, Luisa could now interpret it as a sign of the baby's presence and her signaling her need for care. Using her new skills of visualization, she imagined herself getting closer to that incubator and imagined herself embracing her little baby self and feeling better, any time she wanted.

This session was one of the cornerstones of the work with Luisa. Treatment continued with the processing of various disturbing events in her history. It would take some time before she felt the contact with herself and the parts of her body on a regular basis. Initially, the risk of dissociation was always present in the face of different triggers, but gradually it reduced, allowing her to get more in contact with her body and to attenuate those feelings of loss of meaning and isolation regarding people close to her. Over time, this has allowed her to leave the dangerous relationship and come closer to healthier ones. As often happens for people with these experiences, *normal* relationships are perceived as a pale substitute for the old *more exciting* relationship and there can be a nostalgia for those more intense moments—the illusory call of a lost Eden. This was the price she paid for more stability and much less suffering. The completion of her studies in social services and the following work activity contributed to the strengthening of her ego and to improving Luisa's life.

REFERENCES

Fisher, J. (2017). Trauma-informed stabilisation treatment: A new approach to treating unsafe behaviour. *Australian Clinical Psychologist*, 3(1), 55–62. https://janinafisher.com/pdfs/2017-tist-australian-psychologist.pdf

Hofmann, A. (2009). The Inverted EMDR Standard Protocol for unstable complex post-traumatic stress disorder. In M. Luber (Ed.), *Eye movement desensitization and reprocessing: EMDR scripted protocols: Special populations* (pp. 313–328). Springer Publishing Company.

Jarero, I., Artigas, L., López Cano, T., Mauer, M. & Alcalá, N. (1999, November). *Children's post traumatic stress after natural disasters: Integrative treatment protocol*. Poster presented at the Annual Meeting of the International Society for Traumatic Stress Studies, Miami, FL.

Krupnik, V. (2018). Differential effects of an evolutionary-based EMDR therapy on depression and anxiety symptoms: A case series study. *Journal of EMDR Practice and Research*, 12(2), 46–57. https://doi.org/10.1891/1933-3196.12.2.46

Paulsen, P. D., Sandra, L. & O'Shea, M. S. (2017). *When there are no words: Repairing early trauma and neglect from the attachment period with EMDR therapy*. CreateSpace Independent Publishing Platform.

Future Perspectives of EMDR Therapy

10

The State of Research and Practical Experience on Treating Bipolar Disorder With EMDR Therapy

Benedikt L. Amann

This is the first time that a psychiatrist was interested in everything that has happened in my life.
—Joan, 45 years old, bipolar disorder type I

INTRODUCTION

In this chapter on treating bipolar disorder with eye movement desensitization and reprocessing (EMDR) therapy, expert Benedikt L. Amann discusses the affective spectrum and bipolar disorder specifically. Bipolar disorder is a strongly genetically influenced illness that overlaps with other psychiatric illnesses such as schizoaffective disorders, depression, or psychosis. The etiology of this disorder frequently includes—beyond a polygenetic basis—dysfunctional family background and childhood trauma. There is a high risk for suicide, especially in the depressive and mixed phases of the illness, but, next to medication as the basis for treatment, psychoeducation and psychosocial interventions are helpful. For psychotherapy with these patients, Benedikt L. Amann developed—with his research group—five EMDR subprotocols to be used in EMDR's Phase 2, including a psychotherapeutic mood stabilizer protocol with indications, in a pilot trial, that these patients' moods get better without causing affective relapses during the processing of trauma and adverse life experiences.

WHAT IS BIPOLAR DISORDER?

Mood changes are common in life and occur particularly in the context of stressful situations. The transition from normal mood changes to pathological affect disorders is fluid. The latter must be considered when mood swings have a longer duration and stronger characteristics, and at the same time negatively influence the person's quality of life. Even within affective disorders, there is a meaningful range of variants. In order to be able to define changes in mood better, the term *affective spectrum* was established, a term that ranges from unipolar depression to cyclothymia to bipolar I and bipolar II disorders (Phillips & Kupfer, 2013).

The most well-known of these disorders is bipolar I disorder, which is characterized by strongly pronounced euphoric manias (with an inpatient stay in a psychiatric clinic) and depression alternately. The lifetime prevalence for bipolar I disorder is around 1%. Bipolar II disorder occurs with about the same frequency, characterized by alternating depression and hypomania. Hypomania describes euphoric episodes, but less strongly pronounced and without the necessity of a psychiatric inpatient stay. Bipolar II disorder is often difficult to diagnose, as hypomanic episodes are not correctly identified in patients with unipolar depression. Recurring monopolar hypomania or mania, on the other hand, plays a subordinate role from a clinical perspective. Cyclothymia, which is itself not uncommon, is characterized by regular, more mild hypomania and more mild depressive phases for a period of at least 2 years. However, it does not fulfill the criterion of typical hypomania or depression. Particularly for cyclothymia, it is a very personal decision whether it is necessary to utilize pharmaceutical treatment.

Considering the complete spectrum of bipolar disorders, it is possible to say that around 4 million people in Germany will be affected by a bipolar disorder at least once in their lives. If one limits this to just the typical bipolar I disorder, then it is still approximately 800,000 people. Nonetheless, one must assume that only about 200,000—just a quarter—of affected people will be diagnosed in the most narrow sense of the definition, and that only about 80,000 will be able to be considered adequately treated (German Society for Bipolar Disorders—Deutsche Gesellschaft für Bipolare Störungen e.V, 2003). This is important when one keeps in mind that bipolar patients have an elevated mortality due to a roughly 30 times higher suicide mortality and cardiologic comorbidities, in comparison to the rest of the population (Angst et al., 2002). During manic phases, patients experience an intense exhilaration, enhanced performance and creativity, a considerably lower need for sleep, quick changes from exhilaration to irritability, sexual disinhibition, and have an urge to speak at inappropriate times, which is less pronounced—as described previously—in hypomanic phases. Patients in the depressive phases exhibit symptoms, such as an enhanced feeling of sadness, lack of motivation, lack of interest in things, loss of sexual interest, tendency toward constant rumination, as well as a pessimistic view of the future with suicidal ideation, sleep disturbances, waking up very early or an increased need for sleep, loss of appetite or increased food intake, and disruptions in concentration and attention. In mixed episodes, manic and depressive episodes can occur in rapid alternation or even at the same time. Those affected are agitated or driven while feeling despondent and depressed in equal measure. Precisely because of the combination of increased activity and depression, the suicide risk is particularly high in this form.

Additional important terms in the context of bipolar disorders are the concepts of polarity, rapid cycling, subsyndromal symptoms, and functional impairment. The concept of polarity describes the fact that patients in the course of their bipolar disorder often develop predominantly (hypo)manic episodes or predominantly depressive episodes (Colom et al., 2006). The predominant polarity correspondingly influences the choice of mood stabilizers that will be more effective against depressive or (hypo)manic episodes. Rapid cycling, a temporary state that is often difficult to treat in bipolar patients, is defined by four or more affective episodes per year (Carvalho et al., 2014). In addition to changes in mood, around 40% to 60% of bipolar patients suffer from cognitive deficits and functional losses, with a noticeably reduced quality of life (Bonnin et al., 2019).

In recent years, specific interventions have been developed to improve the functioning level of bipolar patients (Torrent et al., 2013). Additional psychosocial interventions have also been developed, such as psychoeducation, family interventions, interpersonal and social rhythm therapy, schema-focused therapy, or mindfulness (review: Salcedo et al., 2016), that reduce the risk of further episodes by around 15%. In this context, it seems important that this result is largely based on psychoeducational interventions, but that psychosocial interventions are generally insufficiently integrated into the daily care of bipolar patients. It is probably also for this reason that bipolar patients' risk of suffering from an additional affective episode is high overall: 70% of bipolar I patients and almost 80% of bipolar II patients will suffer from at least one additional episode within the next 5 years after an acute depressive or (hypo)manic phase (Radua et al., 2017). Additionally, a clinical remission of affective symptoms is achieved rarely; rather, patients frequently show subsyndromal symptoms, described previously, that in turn represent a clear risk factor for further affective episodes (Radua et al., 2017). It is important to note that a lack of understanding of the illness, as well as insufficient medication compliance, also play large roles. The most frequent psychiatric comorbidities are anxiety disorders (42%), substance abuse (33%), and borderline personality disorder (22%), all of which can potentially worsen the progression of the patient's bipolar disorder (Vieta et al., 2018). In the context of this book, it seems important to mention that posttraumatic stress disorder (PTSD) is also a frequent comorbidity, with an approximate 20% lifetime prevalence for bipolar patients (Hernandez et al., 2013).

ETIOLOGY OF BIPOLAR DISORDER

The development of bipolar disorder is a multifactorial process. In 2021, a large-scale genome-wide association study was published that identified 64 gene loci for bipolar disorder (Mullins et al., 2021). This means that bipolar disorder is an unspecific, polygenetic illness that overlaps with other psychiatric illnesses such as schizoaffective disorders, psychosis, or depression. This genetic predisposition causes changes in neurotransmitters such as serotonin, dopamine, or noradrenaline, cellular signals, molecular transporters, or neurotrophic factors such as brain-derived neurotrophic factor (BDNF). The latter neurotrophic factors, which are responsible for the growth of cells, were investigated in bipolar disorder and in the context of trauma, and it was found that the BDNF is lower for bipolar disorder than it is for the general population, but is even more reduced in the case of a previous psychological trauma (Kauer-Sant'Anna et al., 2007).

In 2012, this led to an exciting hypothesis in a study published in *Molecular Psychiatry* (Rakofsky et al., 2012): Based on the observation that bipolar patients often suffer from a PTSD–bipolar symptom complex, the authors describe that, for patients with childhood trauma, the BDNF is reduced in childhood and there is therefore a greater predisposition for a first depressive episode in adolescence. After another trauma, the BDNF is again reduced, patients are often treated with antidepressants, and this combination can then lead to a first manic phase and a clinically mixed complex of affective and trauma-typical symptoms. As early as 1995, a famous epidemiological study in the United States (Kessler et al., 1995) described that PTSD patients were subject to a five times greater risk of developing a depressive disorder later in the course of their illness. It is interesting to note that the risk (especially for men) that they will suffer a manic episode (i.e., bipolar I disorder) is up to ten times greater than it is for the normal population. This is a result that indicates that childhood trauma plays a role in the etiology of bipolar disorder in the later adult years. This fact, however, is widely ignored in the clinical context even today and was revived only by a 2016 meta-analysis about the role of childhood trauma in later development of bipolar disorder (Palmier-Claus et al., 2016).

A year later, an umbrella review and meta-analysis was published about etiological risk factors for bipolar disorder, with astounding results (Bortolato et al., 2017). The authors analyzed the statistical robustness of risk factors identified in previous meta-analyses for bipolar disorder: asthma, childhood trauma, birth complications, traumatic brain injury, irritable bowel syndrome, obesity, or *Toxoplasma gondii* infection. The two most statistically robust risk factors were irritable bowel syndrome and childhood trauma. Interestingly, there is a correlation between somatic symptom disorders, such as irritable bowel syndrome or fibromyalgia and so on, and psychological trauma (Afari et al., 2014), and for this reason both risk factors indicate that early trauma represents a strong risk factor for suffering later from bipolar disorder. In this context, it should be pointed out that scientific evidence is growing for the fact that childhood traumas overall represent a risk factor for developing each and every psychiatric illness in adolescence or adulthood, and therapeutic options should urgently be established to be able to treat trauma-typical syndromes in the psychiatric context (Rafiq et al., 2018). There is also sufficient scientific evidence showing that childhood traumas leave neuroanatomical traces that then represent the basis for later psychiatric symptoms. In a review in *Nature Review Neuroscience,* Teicher et al. (2016) illustrated which volume reductions, lowered connectivities, and function changes in the brain are caused by which childhood traumas.

TREATMENT OF BIPOLAR DISORDER

Mood stabilizers form the basis of treating bipolar patients. The clinical goal, in terms of the patient, is to improve mood swings without causing bigger side effects. For this purpose, bipolar patients are prescribed different classes of medications, such as lithium salts; anticonvulsants such as valproate, lamotrigine, or carbamazepine; and atypical neuroleptics such as olanzapine, quetiapine, or asenapine. According to the individual profile of each patient that includes their polarity, risk for side effects, and previous experience, mood stabilizers are often recommended in combination. It seems important in this context always to consider the patient's desire, since this automatically improves their compliance. It goes beyond the scope of this chapter to discuss each medication in terms of effects and side effects in the treatment of bipolar disorder. Lithium, a salt, should nonetheless be briefly mentioned here since it has been used for more than 60 years in the treatment of bipolar disorder and continues to represent the most effective medication in bipolar I disorder (Simhandl et al., 2014). Additionally, it is the only medication to have a proven antisuicidal effect.

Chapter 10 Treating Bipolar Disorder With EMDR Therapy

At regular intervals, international treatment recommendations are published for bipolar patients and are based on scientific evidence. Anyone who would like more information can read about various medications, their specific side effect profile, as well as psychotherapeutic interventions, as mentioned in a recently published treatment guideline (Yatham et al., 2018). As described earlier, there are a number of psychosocial/psychotherapeutic interventions for bipolar disorder that have been investigated since the 1990s, which have also become established, more or less, since then. Psychoeducation stands out here and appears to contribute most to relapse prevention among the psychosocial interventions. The problem remains that psychosocial therapies are insufficiently implemented in the everyday routine of clinical patients in general psychiatric wards. This may be connected to insufficient personnel and a lack of training opportunities.

In the context of this book, it is important to mention that there are gaps in the scientific research on therapy. There is a large contrast between scientific evidence for the negative role of psychological trauma and lived experiences in bipolar disorder and therapy options, that have been barely studied (review: Aldinger & Schulze, 2017). To date, there are no established psychotherapeutic interventions that also include trauma-relevant aspects in their complete therapeutic concept for bipolar patients (Landin-Romero et al., 2019).

SCIENTIFIC EVIDENCE AND PRACTICAL EXPERIENCE OF EMDR IN THE TREATMENT OF BIPOLAR DISORDER

Alongside a summary of the scientific status of EMDR in the treatment of bipolar disorder, I also briefly describe stabilization techniques and our overall experience of using EMDR for bipolar disorder. At the beginning of my career, my scientific focus in Munich was centered on clinical pharmacology, primarily pharmacological studies of bipolar disorder. Afterward, in Barcelona, I proceeded to more neurological terrain by studying structural and functional brain changes in psychiatric illnesses, in that case primarily bipolar and schizoaffective disorders. I also began my EMDR training in Barcelona, which not only suddenly facilitated the treatment of my deeply traumatized psychiatric patients' traumas, but also led to a form of exploration and treatment that was more oriented toward the patient's biography and less fixated on psychiatric pathology. Additionally, I found it very helpful that there was now the possibility to strengthen positive resources in my chronic patients with bilateral stimulation (BLS). The patients consistently responded positively to this (see the quote at the beginning of the chapter) and many were able to be stabilized through EMDR.

During my EMDR basic training in Barcelona, BLS in the form of eye movements first left me incredulous, but then quickly fascinated me. Right at the beginning, I had the thought that this represented an elegant mode of access to the brain and could contribute to potential mood stabilization in bipolar patients. It was in this way that my *bipolar grand idea* developed, that EMDR could be a psychotherapeutic mood stabilizer. A hypothesis—to be upfront about it—that has not yet been confirmed in a large randomized and controlled study, since this study is not yet completed at this time (for the study protocol, see Moreno-Alcázar et al., 2017).

The scientific evidence for EMDR for bipolar disorder, like other trauma-oriented processes such as cognitive restructuring (e.g., Mueser et al., 2015), remains in its infancy.

To date, a South Korean case study (Oh & Kim, 2014) and a randomized, controlled pilot study (Novo et al., 2014) about EMDR in bipolar disorder have been published. In the case study, the authors describe two cases of bipolar patients with comorbid PTSD. These were treated with 9, in one case, and 10, in the other, weekly EMDR sessions. After the end of treatment, both patients experienced a remission of trauma-typical symptoms as well as stabilization of their mood, which was maintained after a 1-year follow-up.

In the randomized controlled study of my working group, 20 bipolar I and bipolar II patients with subsyndromal, affective symptoms and a positive trauma history were included and randomized either for individual EMDR therapy (12–16 sessions) or treatment as usual (TAU). All patients were evaluated at the beginning of treatment, after the end of treatment (12 weeks), and in a follow-up (24 weeks). The results showed a statistically significant reduction in affective symptoms (particularly in hypomanic symptoms) in the EMDR group at the end of treatment. Affective symptoms were measured by independent raters using the Hamilton Depression Rating Scale and the Young Mania Rating Scale. However, the results at the 24-week follow-up lost their statistical significance. Regarding trauma symptoms, the Clinician-Administered PTSD Scale and the Impact Event Scale were used, and the results here also showed a statistically significant reduction in the EMDR group at the end of treatment.

In the follow up, a statistically significant reduction was maintained in the Impact Event Scale. Aside from a positive effect of EMDR in subsyndromal bipolar patients with traumas in their history, no side effects and no affective destabilization were observed in this study. The loss of statistical significance, particularly in the follow up, in some scales can probably be understood in light of the small sample of a pilot study.

One of the patients underwent a functional magnet resonance tomography (fMRT) before and after EMDR therapy while being stabilized by medication (Landin-Romero et al., 2013). Here, the n-back test was used, which can measure working memory and also the default mode network (DMN). The DMN represents connected areas of the brain, such as the medial prefrontal cortex, posterior cingulate gyrus, precuneus, medial temporal regions, or the inferior parietal lobule, that are active during inaction or daydreaming and deactivated during a cognitive task. A positive modulation of the DMN is significant, since the tasks of the DMN include introspective thinking, remembering personal events or experiences, social or emotional judgment, imagining the future, and theory of mind tasks. In the future, there will certainly be large-scale fMRT studies of PTSD patients that will investigate brain-specific networks such as the DMN. A *Nature* publication using a mouse model facilitated the first precise neuroanatomical pathways of EMDR (Baek et al., 2019). The superior colliculus mediated persistent attenuation of fear after successfully inducing a lasting reduction in fear in mice by alternating visual bilateral stimulation (AVBS). AVBS yielded sustained increases in the activities of the superior colliculus and mediodorsal thalamus and suppressed the activity of fear-encoding cells and stabilized inhibitory neurotransmission in the basolateral amygdala through a feed-forward inhibitory circuit from the mediodorsal thalamus.

After our controlled study, we developed an EMDR bipolar manual that represents the essence of our first study (Amann et al., 2015). This protocol has been published in M. Luber's book *EMDR Scripted Protocols and Summary Sheets: Treating Anxiety, Obsessive-Compulsive and Mood-Related Conditions* (Amann et al., 2015) and consists of a detailed evaluation of possible traumatic events, five subprotocols in Phase 2 (mood stabilization, improving understanding and compliance, internalizing prodromal symptoms, and de-idealization of manic symptoms), and the Standard EMDR Protocol (Shapiro, 2001) in order to process identified traumas. As described previously, this protocol is currently being investigated in a large randomized study versus supportive psychotherapy in 82 bipolar patients with traumas in their history (Moreno-Alcázar et al., 2017). Patients in both groups receive 20 individual sessions of 60 minutes over a period of 6 months and the goal is to show whether EMDR prevents affective relapses after 12 and 24 months better than supportive psychotherapy does. Additional goals include the improvement of psychiatric symptoms, an improvement of cognition generally, better social cognition, and a higher level of function in the EMDR group.

Currently, a Dutch group is conducting an additional randomized controlled study of 36 bipolar patients with subsyndromal symptoms and trauma in their history to test if the Standard EMDR Protocol improves trauma-associated and affective symptoms (personal communication, Ad de Jongh, 2019).

Altogether, one can say that there is initial scientific evidence that EMDR therapy can be helpful for bipolar patients with traumas in their history. Additionally, there are initial indications that mood gets better for bipolar patients without causing affective relapses during the processing of trauma. Here, it seems important that larger randomized controlled studies are necessary (two studies are currently ongoing) in order to confirm these first results.

PRACTICAL EXPERIENCE AND STABILIZATION TECHNIQUES

From the clinical perspective, it is necessary to explore trauma history in more detail when working with bipolar patients. This includes—alongside possible childhood traumas, bullying, or negative or positive life experiences before affective episodes—psychiatric stays, mechanical restraint, or medication against the will of the patient as well. The idea behind this is that patients are more likely to agree to taking medication and regular psychiatric care when iatrogenic traumas are processed using EMDR. Many bipolar patients are subjected to these incidents or other negative—or also perhaps positive—life events that could affectively destabilize these patients. Therefore, we recommend Hofmann's *Inverted EMDR Standard Protocol* (2009) that facilitates processing traumatic events in the present and then placing these in the context of past experiences.

In our experience, bipolar patients often have complex traumas and therefore require much stabilization. In order to reach the window of tolerance, the methods that have proven themselves best, next to the protocol for the Safe Place, are the Mood Stabilizer Protocol in our EMDR bipolar manual (Amann et al., 2015) and Shapiro's four elements (2009, 2012).

The EMDR Mood Stabilizer Protocol is a short, pragmatic protocol with the aim of installing the situation of a stable mood with the feeling of controlling the patient's life with slow BLS. This is then strengthened with a positive cognition and somatic body representation, again with BLS. Here, I recommend using this protocol at the beginning of every session as a form of a psychotherapeutic mood stabilization.

Working with different parts of the person is also often necessary, due to dissociative symptoms that can impede the processing of experienced traumas. When one offers the patients a therapeutically protective framework, EMDR can be used in bipolar patients to process psychological traumas. Here, the appropriate tools are the Standard EMDR Protocol (Shapiro, 2001) and the EMDR Recent Traumatic Episode Protocol (R-TEP) by Shapiro and Laub (2009), in the case of a recent traumatic episode.

Case Study 10.1

DIAGNOSIS AND TREATMENT OF A YOUNG FEMALE WITH EMDR THERAPY

The female patient is 27 years old and was sent to us from another psychiatric hospital with the question of whether she had a bipolar disorder. The diagnoses at referral to our subacute ward (where up to a 3-month stay is possible) were borderline personality disorder and polytoxicomania, currently abstinent. Medications at admittance were oxcarbazepine as a mood stabilizer, topiramate for impulsivity, and clonazepam for anxiety symptoms. During the first 2 weeks, the patient had labile affect, alternating from ultra-rapid cycling to 2- to 3-day depressive episodes to clearly hypomanic symptoms. She also indicated suffering from auditory hallucinations, although these could be best interpreted in terms of a dissociative experience. The patient, who also exhibited racist thoughts, was ambivalent from the very beginning about her voluntary inpatient stay, and for this reason a therapeutic plan had to be developed rapidly. Here, an important element was the history taking, in which the patient reported having been a happy child until age 6. Then, her father began prolonged systematic psychological and sexual abuse that lasted until she was 13 and was confirmed by her mother, when asked to report her daughter's history separately.

At age 10, she starting self-harming behavior in connection with negative thinking; 3 years later, she started regularly consuming cocaine and cannabis. By 13, she became involved with a bad crowd from the drug world. At 16, she developed severe mood swings, irritability, impulsivity, auditory hallucinations, and anorexia then bulimia. In spite of this, she continued to get good grades in school and she completed her secondary education and began her university studies majoring in simultaneous interpretation. She stopped consuming drugs of her own volition when she was 23. After a severe car accident at 26, she developed a major depression for the first time and had to be hospitalized, followed by outpatient treatment. It was in the outpatient setting where she first reported her traumatic childhood to a psychologist, and she had three EMDR sessions. Several months later, she was transferred to my unit, due to her severe mood swings.

During the Stabilization Phase, at week 1, I changed two of her medications: instead of oxcarbazepine, I prescribed valproate, a different mood stabilizer, and instead of clonazepam, I prescribed a low dose of quetiapine, due to a persisting sleep disturbance. Topiramate was retained. I also installed a Safe Place with the patient and used our EMDR Mood Stabilizer Protocols. Then, we were able to process psychological and sexual abuse by her father in three sessions with the Standard EMDR Protocol. This took up an additional week. After 2 weeks, the patient was euthymic, without impulsivity, auditory hallucinations, or anxieties. Interestingly, she no longer considered herself a racist. As part of a "self-care process," she was able to end her toxic, significant relationship. After staying a few nights at home, her mother noted a positive change in her. After 4 weeks, the patient was discharged from her inpatient stay and begin outpatient psychiatric and EMDR treatment. Her stable condition remained at her follow-up 2 years after discharge.

REFERENCES

Afari, N., Ahumada, S. M., Wright, L. J., Mostoufi, S., Golnari, G., Reis, V., & Cuneo, J. G. (2014). Psychological trauma and functional somatic syndromes: A systematic review and meta-analysis. *Psychosomatic Medicine, 76*(1), 2–11. https://doi.org/10.1097/PSY.0000000000000010

Aldinger, F., & Schulze, T. G. (2017). Environmental factors, life events, and trauma in the course of bipolar disorder. *Psychiatry Clinical Neurosciences, 71*(1), 6–17. https://doi.org/10.1111/pcn.12433

Amann, B. L., Batalla, R., Blanch, V., Capellades, D., Carvajal, M. J., Fernández, I., García, F., Lupo, W., Ponte, M., Sánchez, J., Sanfiz, J., Santed, A., & Luber, M. (2015). The EMDR therapy protocol for bipolar disorder. In M. Luber (Ed.), *Eye movement desensitization and reprocessing (EMDR) scripted protocols and summary sheets: Treating trauma, anxiety and mood-related conditions* (pp. 223–287). Springer Publishing Company.

Angst, F., Stassen, H. H., Clayton, P. J. & Angst, J. (2002). Mortality of patients with mood disorders: Follow-up over 34–38 years. *Journal of Affective Disorders, 68*(2–3), 167–181. https://doi.org/10.1016/s0165-0327(01)00377-9

Baek, J., Lee, S., Cho, T., Kim, S. W., Kim, M., Yoon, Y., Kim, K. K., Byun, J., Kim, S. J., Jeong, J., & Shin, H. S. (2019, February). Neural circuits underlying a psychotherapeutic regimen for fear disorders. *Nature, 566*(7744), 339–343. https://doi.org/10.1038/s41586-019-0931-y

Bonnín, C. D. M., Reinares, M., Martínez-Arán, A., Jiménez, E., Sánchez-Moreno, J., Solé, B., Montejo, L., & Vieta, E. (2019). Improving functioning, quality of life, and well-being in patients with bipolar disorder. *International Journal Neuropsychopharmacology, 22*(8), 467–477. https://doi.org/10.1093/ijnp/pyz018

Bortolato, B., Köhler, C. A., Evangelou, E., León-Caballero, J., Solmi, M., Stubbs, B., Belbasis, L., Pacchiarotti, I., Kessing, L. V., Berk, M. Vieta, E., & Carvalho, A. F. (2017). Systematic assessment of environmental risk factors for bipolar disorder: An umbrella review of systematic reviews and meta-analyses. *Bipolar Disorders, 19*(2), 84–96. https://doi.org/10.1111/bdi.12490

Carvalho, A. F., Dimellis, D., Gonda, X., Vieta, E., McIntyre, R. S., & Fountoulakis, K. N. (2014). Rapid cycling in bipolar disorder: A systematic review. *Journal of Clinical Psychiatry, 75*(6), e578–586. https://doi.org/10.4088/JCP.13r08905

Colom, F., Vieta, E., Daban, C., Pacchiarotti, I., & Sánchez-Moreno, J. (2006, July). Clinical and therapeutic implications of predominant polarity in bipolar disorder. *Journal of Affective Disorders, 93*(1–3), 13–17. https://doi.org/10.1016/j.jad.2006.01.032

Deutsche Gesellschaft für Bipolare Störungen e.V. (2003). *Weißbuch bipolare Störungen in Deutschland*. Books on Demand GmbH.

Hernandez, J. M., Cordova, M. J., Ruzek, J., Reiser, R., Gwizdowski, I. S., Suppes, T., & Ostacher, M. J. (2013). Presentation and prevalence of PTSD in a bipolar disorder population: A STEP-BD examination. *Journal of Affective Disorders, 150*(2), 450–455. https://doi.org/10.1016/j.jad.2013.04.038

Hofmann, A. (2009). The Inverted EMDR Standard Protocol for unstable complex post-traumatic stress disorder. In M. Luber (Ed.), *Eye movement desensitization and reprocessing: EMDR scripted protocols: Special populations* (pp. 313–328). Springer Publishing Company.

Kauer-Sant'Anna, M., Tramontina, J., Andreazza, A. C., Cereser, K., da Costa, S., Santin, A., Yatham, L. N., & Kapczinski, F. (2007). Traumatic life events in bipolar disorder: Impact on BDNF levels and psychopathology. *Bipolar Disorders, 9*(Suppl 1), 128–135. https://doi.org/10.1111/j.1399-5618.2007.00478.x

Kessler, R. C., Sonnega, A., Bromet, E., Hughes, M., & Nelson, C. B. (1995, December). Posttraumatic stress disorder in the National Comorbidity Survey. *Archives of General Psychiatry, 52*(12), 1048–1060. https://doi.org/10.1001/archpsyc.1995.03950240066012

Landin-Romero, R., Novo, P., Santed, A., Vicens, V., Pomarol-Clotet, E., McKenna, P., Salgado, P., Shapiro, F., & Amann, B. L. (2013). Clinical and brain functional improvement in a bipolar patient with subsyndromal mood symptoms following EMDR therapy. *Neuropsychobiology, 67*(3), 181–184. https://doi.org/10.1159/000346654

Landin-Romero, R., Moreno-Alcázar, A., Ferguson, G., Pérez, V., & Amann, B. L. (2019, May). That which does not kill you—May afflict you? Psychological trauma in bipolar disorder. *Bipolar Disorders*, *21*(3), 192–193. https://doi.org/10.1111/bdi.12766

Moreno-Alcázar, A., Radua, J., Landín-Romero, R., Blanco, L., Madre, M., Reinares, M., Comes, M., Jiménez, E., Crespo, J. M., Vieta, E., Pérez, V., Novo, P., Doñate, M., Cortizo, R., Valiente-Gómez, A., Lupo, W., McKenna, P. J., Pomarol-Clotet, E., & Amann, B. L. (2017). Eye movement desensitization and reprocessing therapy versus supportive therapy in affective relapse prevention in bipolar patients with a history of trauma: Study protocol for a randomized controlled trial. *Trials*, *18*(1), Article 160. https://doi.org/10.1186/s13063-017-1910-y

Mueser, K. T., Gottlieb, J. D., Xie, H., Lu, W., Yanos, P. T., Rosenberg, S. D., Silverstein, S. M., Duva, S. M., Minsky, S., Wolfe, R. S., & McHugo, G. J. (2015). Evaluation of cognitive restructuring for post-traumatic stress disorder in people with severe mental illness. *British Journal of Psychiatry*, *206*(6), 501–508. https://doi.org/10.1192/bjp.bp.114.147926

Mullins, N., Forstner, A. J., O'Connell, K. S., Coombes, B., Coleman, J. R. I., Qiao, Z., Als, T. D., Bigdeli, T. B., Børte, S., Bryois, J., Charney, A. W., Drange, O. K., Gandal, M. J., Hagenaars, S. P., Ikeda, M., Kamitaki, N., Kim, M., Krebs, K., Panagiotaropoulou, G., ... Andreassen, O. A. (2021, June). Genome-wide association study of more than 40,000 bipolar disorder cases provides new insights into the underlying biology. *Nature Genetics*, *53*(6), 817–829. https://doi.org/10.1038/s41588-021-00857-4

Novo, P., Landin, R., Radua, J., Vicens, V., McKenna, P., Pomarol-Clotet, E., Fernandez, I., Garcia, F., Shapiro, F., & Amann, B. L. (2014). EMDR as add-on to pharmacological treatment in subsyndromal, bipolar patients with a history of traumatic events: A randomized, single-blind, controlled pilot-study. *Psychiatry Research*, *219*(1), 122–128. https://doi.org/10.1016/j.psychres.2014.05.012

Oh, D., & Kim, D. (2014). Eye movement desensitization and reprocessing for posttraumatic stress disorder in bipolar disorder. *Psychiatry Investigation*, *11*(3), 340–341. https://doi.org/10.4306/pi.2014.11.3.340

Palmier-Claus, J. E., Berry, K., Bucci, S., Mansell, W., & Varese, F. (2016). Relationship between childhood adversity and bipolar affective disorder: Systematic review and meta-analysis. *British Journal of Psychiatry*, *209*(6), 454–459. https://doi.org/10.1192/bjp.bp.115.179655

Phillips, M. L., & Kupfer, D. J. (2013). Bipolar disorder diagnosis: Challenges and future directions. *The Lancet*, *11*, *381*(9878), 1663–1671. https://doi.org/10.1016/S0140-6736(13)60989-7

Rafiq, S., Campodonico, C., & Varese, F. (2018). The relationship between childhood adversities and dissociation in severe mental illness: A meta-analytic review. *Acta Psychiatrica Scandinavica*, *138*(6), 509–525. https://doi.org/10.1111/acps.12969

Rakofsky, J. J., Ressler, K. J., & Dunlop, B. W. (2012, January). BDNF function as a potential mediator of bipolar disorder and post-traumatic stress disorder comorbidity. *Molecular Psychiatry*, *17*(1), 22–35. https://doi.org/10.1038/mp.2011.121

Radua, J., Grunze, H., & Amann, B. L. (2017). Meta-analysis of the risk of relapse in bipolar disorder. *Psychotherapy and Psychosomatics*, *86*(2), 90–98. https://doi.org/10.1159/000449417

Salcedo, S., Gold, A. K., Sheikh, S., Marcus, P. H., Nierenberg, A. A., Deckersbach, T., & Sylvia, L. G. (2016). Empirically supported psychosocial interventions for bipolar disorder: Current state of the research. *Journal of Affective Disorders*, *1*(201), 203–214. https://doi.org/10.1016/j.jad.2016.05.018

Shapiro, E. (2009). Four elements exercise for stress management. In M. Luber (Ed.), *Eye movement desensitization and reprocessing (EMDR) scripted protocols: Basics and special situations* (pp. 73–79). Springer Publishing Company.

Shapiro, E. (2012). *4 elements exercises for stress reduction (earth-air-water-fire)*. EMDR Foundation. https://emdrfoundation.org/toolkit/four-elements.pdf

Shapiro, E., & Laub, B. (2009). The recent-traumatic episode protocol (R-TEP): An integrative protocol for early EMDR intervention (EEI). In M. Luber (Ed.), *Eye movement desensitization and* reprocessing (EMDR) scripted protocols: Basics and special situations (pp. 251–269). Springer Publishing Company.

Shapiro, F. (2001). *Eye movement desensitization and reprocessing: Basic principles, protocols, and procedures* (2nd ed.). [Internet]. Guilford Press.

Simhandl, C., König, B., & Amann, B. L. (2014) A prospective 4 year naturalistic follow-up of treatment and outcome of 300 bipolar I and II patients. *Journal of Clinical Psychiatry, 3,* 254–262. https://doi.org/10.4088/JCP.13m08601

Teicher, M. H., Samson, J. A., Anderson, C. M., & Ohashi, K. (2016). The effects of childhood maltreatment on brain structure, function and connectivity. *Nature Reviews Neuroscience, 17*(10), 652–666. https://doi.org/10.1038/nrn.2016.111

Torrent, C., del Mar Bonnin, C., Martínez-Arán, A., Valle, J., Amann, B. L., González-Pinto, A., Crespo, J. M., Ibáñez, Á., Garcia-Portilla, M. P., Tabarés-Seisdedos, R., Arango, C., Colom, F., Solé, B., Pacchiarotti, I., Rosa, A. R., Ayuso-Mateos, J. L., Anaya, C., Fernández, P., Landín-Romero, R., ... Vieta, E. (2013). Efficacy of functional remediation in bipolar disorder: A multicenter, randomized controlled study. *American Journal of Psychiatry, 170*(8), 852–859. https://doi.org/10.1176/appi.ajp.2012.12070971

Vieta, E., Berk, M, Schulze, T. G., Carvalho, A. F., Suppes, T., Calabrese, J. R., Gao, K., Miskowiak, K. W., & Grande, I. (2018). Bipolar disorders. *Nature Reviews Disease Primers, 8*(4), 18008. https://doi.org/10.1038/nrdp.2018.8

Yatham, L. N., Kennedy, S. H., Parikh, S. V., Schaffer, A., Bond, D. J., Frey, B. N., Sharma, V., Goldstein, B. I., Rej, S., Beaulieu, S., Alda, M., MacQueen, G., Milev, R. V., Ravindran, A., O'Donovan, C., McIntosh, D., Lam, R. W., Vazquez, G., Kapczinski F., ... Berk, M. (2018, March). Canadian Network for Mood and Anxiety Treatments (CANMAT) and International Society for Bipolar Disorders (ISBD) 2018 guidelines for the management of patients with bipolar disorder. *Bipolar Disorders, 20*(2), 97–170. https://doi.org/10.1111/bdi.12609

11

Traumatic Events and Severe Recurrent and Chronic Depression and EMDR Therapy: Clinical and Biological Issues

Alessandra Minelli and Elisabetta Maffioletti

INTRODUCTION

Major depressive disorder (MDD) is a disabling psychiatric condition and, although drug treatment is most widely used to treat MDD, drugs are often ineffective and can lead to treatment-resistant depression (TRD) when they do not work. Childhood and adolescent trauma, as well as early adverse life experiences, especially interpersonal traumas/attachment adversity, are risk factors for depression. The biological bases of MDD are explored, including the effect of traumatic and stressful events on gene expression. For example, there is evidence for traumas that occur during early childhood inducing alterations in the stress response system that continue into adulthood, as well as early life adversity affecting molecular pathways relevant to the development of MDD. This suggests that interpersonal traumas like emotional abuse and neglect strongly impact these patients. The expert authors report on studies that show that eye movement desensitization and reprocessing (EMDR) is very effective in improving depressive symptomatology in treatment-resistant MDD patients with a history of trauma.

MAJOR DEPRESSIVE DISORDER: CHRONICITY, RECURRENCE, AND RESISTANCE

MDD is a disabling psychiatric condition leading to a persistent feeling of sadness and loss of interest and it is among the top five leading causes of disability and disease burden throughout the world (Gabilondo et al., 2010; Hasin et al., 2018).

The course of MDD is quite variable; indeed, some patients never, or only rarely, reach remission, considered as a period of at least 2 months without symptoms, or one or two symptoms present in mild severity, whereas others live many years with few or no symptoms between different episodes. The chronicity of the pathology reduces drastically the probability of a complete resolution of the symptomatology. The likelihood of chronic depressive symptoms is substantially increased when there is a combination of personality, anxiety, and substance use disorders.

Moreover, although MDD may occur only once during life, people typically have multiple depressive episodes: In this case, the disease is defined as recurrent depression. For the definition of recurrence, there must be an interval of at least 2 consecutive months between separate episodes in which the criteria for a major depressive episode are not met. At least three quarters of those affected by a first depressive episode will have another during the rest of their lives.

The most widespread therapeutic approach for MDD is drug treatment. Drug therapy helps to improve mood, reduces mental rumination, and alleviates the acute symptoms of the disease. Drugs of different pharmacological types are available and it is the psychiatrist's responsibility to suggest the most suitable therapy for each individual patient. In the first instance, the treatment proposed to the patient is an antidepressant therapy. The most commonly used classes of drugs are the serotonin reuptake inhibitors (SSRIs) and the serotonin and norepinephrine reuptake inhibitors (SNRIs) because of their widely demonstrated efficacy and good tolerability. Tricyclics (TCAs) and other antidepressants such as trazodone, mirtazapine, and vortioxetine are also used. In addition to treatment with antidepressants, in more severe forms and/or in the event of poor or inadequate response to antidepressant treatment alone, other categories of drugs such as antipsychotics (in particular the second-generation ones), mood stabilizers, and benzodiazepines are used in combination.

However, despite all these drugs available for treating MDD, pharmacological therapy alone is often ineffective. The most important pharmacological trials carried out on MDD patients revealed that only about one third of patients respond to the first treatment with antidepressants (Trivedi et al., 2006). Most patients with MDD need different pharmacological treatments, often in combination, to achieve remission of symptoms, and a high percentage of them, about 30% to 40%, are defined as suffering from TRD (Berlim & Turecki, 2007; Thomas et al., 2013). TRD is commonly defined as the failure of treatment to produce response or remission for patients after two or more treatment attempts of adequate dose and duration, but no clear consensus exists about this definition. As a result, the absence of a standardized method to classify TRD causes difficulties in estimating its prevalence.

In MDD, several clinical characteristics have been associated to a chronic course with a higher probability of a negative treatment outcome. These features, often defined as negative clinical predictors, include greater symptom severity, longer duration of an episode, a larger number of episodes, comorbidity, earlier onset, higher neuroticism, life stress events, and childhood adversity (Hasin et al., 2018; Kautzky et al., 2019; Penninx et al., 2011).

THE ROLE OF CHILDHOOD TRAUMA AND STRESSFUL LIFE EVENTS FOR CHRONICITY OF DEPRESSION

It has been widely demonstrated that trauma, particularly when experienced during childhood and adolescence, increases the risk of developing MDD (Nelson et al., 2017;

Poole et al., 2017). Childhood adversities can include sexual, physical, and emotional abuse; neglect; separation from a parent; or mental illness in a parent. Childhood trauma may exert deleterious effects on the development of children and adolescents, with long-term consequences that often persist in adulthood (Mandelli et al., 2015).

Moreover, evidence indicates that traumatic experiences could be associated, directly or indirectly, with a treatment-resistant and chronic, endophenotype of depression (Negele et al., 2015; Williams et al., 2016). Indeed, several studies have shown that stressful life events, including both physical and emotional abuse, are associated with the main and more relevant negative clinical predictors reported, such as earlier illness onset, greater severity of symptoms, presence of psychotic symptoms, suicidal behaviors, and comorbidities (Dias de Mattos Souza et al., 2016; Gaudiano & Zimmerman, 2010; Nelson et al., 2017; Tunnard et al., 2014).

For decades, most research has focused on physical and sexual abuse as risk factors for MDD, whereas fewer studies have examined the effects of other types of abuse and neglect. However, two recent meta-analyses have clearly demonstrated that neglect and emotional abuse, often called *interpersonal traumas* or *attachment adversity*, exert the strongest effect on the development of depression in adulthood (Infurna et al., 2016; Mandelli et al., 2015). The data obtained in these studies are consistent with current results reported in the literature. Indeed, several authors have argued that emotional abuse and neglect in childhood, that typically include experiences of being rejected, degraded, terrorized, isolated, or teased, might be more strongly related to internalizing symptoms and to the development of depression than physical abuse or sexual abuse. Moreover, results have shown that a history of emotional neglect and psychological abuse can predict comorbidity and chronicity in adults with depression. This form of abuse is harder to identify because, in contrast to physical abuse, the marks are left on the inside instead of the outside. Nonetheless, it is important to pay adequate attention during the assessment of traumatic experiences during clients' lives, since all new findings clearly highlight the potentially strong impact of the more *silent* types of childhood maltreatment on the development of depression.

MOLECULAR MECHANISMS RELATED TO MAJOR DEPRESSIVE DISORDER AND TRAUMATIC EVENTS

The biological bases underlying the relationship between the occurrence of life's adversities and the development of severe forms of MDD later in life are still largely unexplained. The first studies conducted to explore this field have suggested that alterations in the way DNA activates or *expresses* itself are at play. The regulation of the expression of genes, that is, the functional units containing the instructions to build proteins, located along the DNA, is fundamental for every biological process. If we consider the different cell types in a multicellular organism, we can observe how they dramatically differ in both structure and function. Compare, for example, a mammalian neuron to a lymphocyte; the differences are so extreme that it is difficult to imagine that the two cells contain the same genome. For this reason, and since cell differentiation is often irreversible, biologists originally suspected that genes were selectively lost during cell differentiation. Today, we know that cell differentiation depends on changes in gene expression, that is, in their activation/deactivation, rather than on changes in the sequence of DNA. Genes are *activated* during transcription, the process by which DNA is copied, or transcribed, to messenger RNA, the molecule that will be subsequently *read* to make proteins. Reflective of its importance for cell survival and function, the regulatory mechanisms controlling gene expression are exquisitely sophisticated (Alberts et al., 2002).

Studies aimed at exploring disease-related alterations in gene expression are classified according to two main approaches: gene studies or transcriptomic studies. As suggested by the name, candidate gene studies focus on one or a few *candidates*, chosen based on an *a priori* hypothesis, for example, because of their role in mechanisms related to the pathology under investigation. On the contrary, through transcriptomic studies, all the transcribed genes are tested. Therefore, this is a hypothesis-free approach.

In MDD, and many other diseases, altered patterns of gene expression have been identified both in the affected organ (concerning MDD, the central nervous system [CNS]) and in peripheral tissues such as the blood. It is important to note that brain and blood cells share about 80% of the transcribed genes. Even if it is still not completely clear to what extent peripheral modifications in gene expression directly reflect brain alterations in CNS diseases, peripheral blood profiling gives researchers the opportunity to study some of the aspects of brain functioning in the absence of human neural tissue. This overcomes the limitations intrinsic to postmortem studies, in parallel with the possibility of exploring systemic or purely peripheral alterations linked to the investigated pathology.

Concerning MDD, alterations in the expression of several genes have been described in both the brain and the blood. Collectively, the genes dysregulated in the brain are mainly implicated in the GABAergic, glutamatergic, and serotonergic neurotransmission. The expression of GABAergic and glutamatergic genes is especially modified in prefrontal cortical areas, which are well known to be involved in mood regulation and depression. Another group of consistently replicated genes are those from the serotonergic family that have been observed as dysregulated predominantly in the dorsolateral prefrontal cortex and in the hippocampus (Ciobanu et al., 2016). In the blood, the identified genes are primarily related to inflammation and immunity, with an enrichment for interleukin-6 signaling and natural killer cell pathways, consistent with the hypothesis that a bidirectional reinforcing communication between the brain and the immune system is part of the disease etiology (Jansen et al., 2016).

In addition to coding genes, modifications in the expression of non-coding RNAs known as microRNAs (or "miRNAs") have been implicated in MDD. Since their discovery in the early 1990s, microRNAs have revolutionized our understanding of gene regulation: they act as posttranscriptional regulators of gene expression by binding to target messenger RNAs, altering their stability and/or inhibiting the subsequent process of translation, that is, the synthesis of proteins. These small but powerful molecules have been shown to play key roles in basic neural functions and in different neurological and psychiatric disorders. Besides their production in cells, microRNAs are released in several body fluids, including peripheral blood, and they can cross the blood–brain barrier. MDD-related alterations in the circulating levels of these molecules have been described by several studies, suggesting an implication of microRNAs involved in pathways that have been already related to MDD, such as different signaling pathways, mainly involved in neurodevelopmental and neurotrophic processes (Ferrúa et al., 2019).

Traumatic events, especially when experienced early in life, have been shown to induce critical changes in gene expression also. Since the early phases of life represent critical moments for the development of brain function, and are characterized by extensive neuroplasticity, they are particularly sensitive to remodeling induced by environmental stimuli. In the case of exposure to adverse events, these can *reprogram* brain development through the regulation of gene expression and determine a negative imprinting that may persist during later stages, possibly until adulthood. According to some authors, adverse experiences could represent *hidden wounds* with an effect comparable, at least in part, to that of physical traumas; many of the physiological responses induced by trauma and psychological stress, such as inflammatory activation, are the same as those caused by physical insults (Danese & van Harmelen, 2017).

In recent years, biomedical research has increasingly focused on the study of the molecular processes mediating the negative effects of trauma on psychological health. Besides the study of gene expression, particular interest was aroused by epigenetic mechanisms. These processes can regulate the expression of genes through chemical modifications of the DNA, mainly consisting of the addition of methyl and acetyl groups directly to the DNA or to histones (the proteins around which the DNA is wrapped). Several studies have shown that traumatic and stressful events can induce epigenetic modifications, therefore affecting gene expression. Moreover, it is particularly interesting to note that when traumas occur in parents before conception or in the mother during the prenatal period, they can have repercussions for the health and behavior of the offspring, in some cases even into subsequent generations. At least for certain types of traumas, the role of mediator between the traumatic event and the phenotype of the descendants seems to be a result of epigenetic alterations, since these are observed in both parents and children. By determining changes to the DNA, epigenetic modifications could directly transmit the effects of adverse events experienced by the parents to the offspring. However, an alternative explanation is that epigenetic changes could be established *de novo* at each generation, as a consequence of the behavioral patterns shown by the person who suffered the trauma. An example could be of living with parents who suffer from trauma-based pathological conditions and transmit this to a next generation via a kind of secondary traumatization.

Many of the studies investigating the effects of trauma on gene expression and epigenetic modifications have employed a candidate gene approach, focusing on major players in the activity of the hypothalamic–pituitary–adrenal (HPA) axis. The interest in this system stems from the fact that it is the main modulator of the adaptation to stress. In the presence of a stressful stimulus, the hypothalamus recognizes the danger and releases the corticotropin-releasing factor (CRF); this hormone induces, in turn, the release of the adrenocorticotropic hormone from the pituitary gland and this targets both the adrenal cortex, that produces glucocorticoids (especially cortisol), and the adrenal medulla, that produces adrenaline. This chain of events helps the body to face dangerous situations, supporting *fight or flight* responses. When the triggering event ceases, the activity of the HPA axis is deactivated by the negative feedback mediated by cortisol. The dysregulation of the HPA axis is a common feature in psychiatric disorders such as anxiety disorders and MDD (McGowan & Matthews, 2018).

Candidate gene studies on the HPA axis concerned, among others, the *nuclear receptor subfamily 3 group C member 1* (*NR3C1*), coding for the glucocorticoid receptor. An increase in the methylation of the promoter of *NR3C1*, associated with a decrease in the expression of this gene, was observed in the brains of people who died by suicide with experiences of childhood maltreatment, compared to those who had not experienced such events (McGowan & Szyf, 2010). This suggests that traumas occurring during early life are able to induce alterations in the stress response system that may persist into adulthood. Similarly, an increase in the NR3C1 promoter methylation, accompanied by decreased gene expression, was observed in adult MDD patients with a history of childhood trauma (Watkeys et al., 2018). In addition to studies focusing on genes related to the HPA axis, other ones used a genome-wide approach to investigate the effects of trauma and stressful events on all the methylated sites of the genome (methylome). By studying the methylome in people with a history of childhood trauma, differentially methylated sites were detected in the promoters of different genes involved in cellular processes related to development (Suderman et al., 2014) and neural plasticity (Labonté et al., 2012).

Traumatic experiences have been also shown to induce alterations in the expression of microRNAs, as recently shown by two studies that reported reduced levels of miR-125b-1-3p and enhanced levels of miR-15a in the blood of adult subjects exposed to childhood trauma. These microRNAs are involved in the control of neurodevelopmental processes and stress response, respectively (Cattane et al., 2019; Volk et al., 2016).

However, despite the several studies conducted on gene and microRNA expression in MDD and the first indications about an involvement of disrupted gene regulation in trauma and stress, the peculiar effects of adverse experiences in MDD patients have been poorly investigated. The regulation of gene expression, especially through microRNAs, has also emerged as a biological mechanism mediating the association between early life adversities and the development of MDD later in life. In a recent study, data on expression of all the genes (transcriptome) and microRNAs (miRNome) in adult rats exposed to prenatal stress were compared with the transcriptomic profiles of healthy subjects exposed to early life stress. Three genes that were involved in biological pathways related to inflammation/immunity and stress response (cytokine, TGF-β1, and glucocorticoid receptor signaling) were identified as dysregulated. Genetic variants in these genes also showed significant interactions with early life emotional stress in predicting depressive symptoms during adulthood (Cattaneo et al., 2018). A handful of studies examined the peripheral expression of a few candidate genes related to the activity of the HPA axis and to inflammation, neurodevelopment, and neurotransmission, and showed an effect of the aggregate expression of a few genes in mediating the relationship between childhood maltreatment and MDD (Bustamante et al., 2016; Spindola et al., 2017). The only available genome-wide findings come from a study conducted on a large RNA sequencing dataset that highlighted a dysregulation of the pro-inflammatory system in MDD patients with a history of emotional abuse during childhood. In the same study, an alteration in the expression of the genes MED22 and ZNF554, both involved in the regulation of transcription, was observed in patients who experienced childhood neglect (Minelli et al., 2018). Overall, these results demonstrate that early life adversity can affect molecular pathways relevant to the development of MDD and suggest that interpersonal traumas such as emotional abuse and neglect exert the strongest impact in MDD patients. There is consistent clinical data that indicate this kind of trauma as the most significant factor associated with depression (Infurna et al., 2016; Mandelli et al., 2015).

Finally, preliminary evidence indicated possible consequences of therapies on gene regulation, exerted by both pharmacological and non-pharmacological treatments (Belzeaux et al., 2018; Kéri et al., 2014; Kolshus et al., 2017); however, so far, these studies have focused on general approaches to treat MDD, without a precise concentration on trauma-focused therapies that specifically address the effects of trauma in MDD patients, such as trauma-focused cognitive behavioral therapy (TF-CBT) and EMDR. These therapies have demonstrated their effectiveness in improving depressive symptomatology in treatment-resistant MDD patients with a history of trauma (Minelli et al., 2019). This study showed that 22 TRD patients (10 treated with TF-CBT and 12 with EMDR) had a reduction in depressive symptomatology, with a greater efficacy for EMDR. The most significant result was that EMDR was as effective as TF-CBT in reducing depression symptoms in TRD patients during hospitalization; however, at the follow-up visit, only EMDR maintained this amelioration.

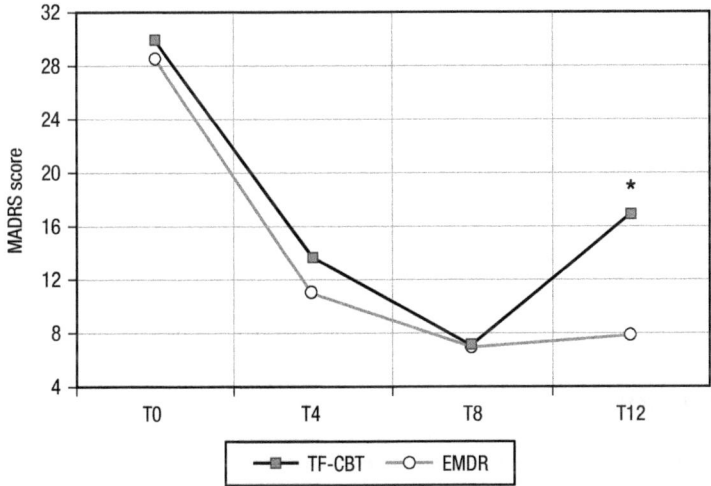

FIGURE 11.1 Course of depressive symptomatology (third-party assessment) during treatment and follow-up in 22 patients treated with EMDR versus trauma-centered behavior therapy.

EMDR, eye movement desensitization and reprocessing; MADRS, Montgomery–Åsberg Depression Rating Scale; TF-CBT, trauma-focused cognitive behavioral therapy.

Source: Minelli, A., Zampieri, E., Sacco, C., Bazzanella, R., Mezzetti, N., Tessari, E., Barlati, S., & Bortolomasi, M. (2019). Clinical efficacy of trauma-focused psychotherapies in treatment-resistant depression (TRD) in-patients: A randomized, controlled pilot-study. *Psychiatry Research, 273*, 567–574. https://doi.org/10.1016/j.psychres.2019.01.070

The Montgomery–Åsberg Depression Rating Scale (MADRS; Figure 11.1) and the Beck Depression Inventory, Second Edition (BDI-II; Figure 11.2), revealed that there was complete agreement between clinicians' and patients' perspectives. In addition, the same pattern of results was obtained when the mood, cognitive, and neurovegetative symptoms were separately analyzed. Interestingly, for neurovegetative symptoms, there was a treatment effect in favor of EMDR that supports the well-documented effect of EMDR in the reduction of hyperarousal activation in severe TRD patients. The amelioration was partly maintained for a long time; indeed, several patients were still in remission after 24 weeks. Comparing the percentages of relapse after 4 months posttreatment, a higher frequency was observed in the TF-CBT group, compared to the EMDR one (50% vs. 25%), although this difference was not statistically significant.

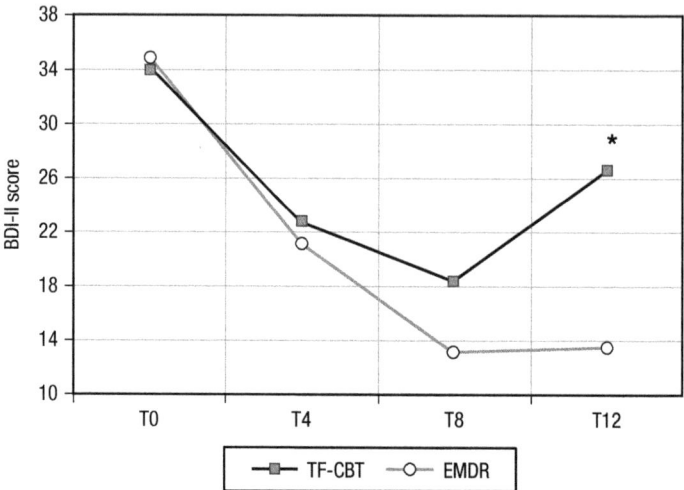

FIGURE 11.2 Course of depressive symptomatology (third-party assessment) during treatment and follow-up in 22 patients treated with EMDR versus trauma-centered behavior therapy.

BDI-II, Beck Depression Inventory, Second Edition; EMDR, eye movement desensitization and reprocessing; TF-CBT, trauma-focused cognitive behavioral therapy.

Source: Minelli, A., Zampieri, E., Sacco, C., Bazzanella, R., Mezzetti, N., Tessari, E., Barlati, S., & Bortolomasi, M. (2019). Clinical efficacy of trauma-focused psychotherapies in treatment-resistant depression (TRD) in-patients: A randomized, controlled pilot-study. *Psychiatry Research, 273*, 567–574. https://doi.org/10.1016/j.psychres.2019.01.070

CONCLUSION

Early traumatic experiences, in particular interpersonal traumas, are linked to a greater risk of developing MDD in adulthood. Childhood traumas in MDD patients are associated with different kinds of biological dysregulation. Although, to date, most studies have focused on the inflammatory system, the results obtained underline the strong impact exerted by childhood traumatic experiences, suggesting that more pervasive effects could be at play. Consequently, it is possible to suppose that the increased risk to develop depression in adulthood could be mediated by a dysregulation in various biological pathways. Moreover, some researchers are investigating if the consequences of traumas experienced by a parent could persist in subsequent generations through epigenetic effects, on the basis of preliminary evidence from animal models. However, it is still unclear what is the weight of a *true* epigenetic transmission of the effects of traumas to subsequent generations and what is instead the influence of the pathological relational environment, potentially capable of inducing *de novo* epigenetic modifications in each generation. Further studies are also warranted to investigate the effects of trauma-focused therapies, with particular relevance for development of future clinical applications. From a clinical point of view, the clarification of the molecular mechanisms that mediate the relationship between early life adversity and MDD could pave the way to preventive and therapeutic possibilities. First, an early estimation of the extent of biological impairment associated with traumatic experiences could offer the opportunity to identify the subjects most at risk of developing mental illness(es) later in life, allowing to plan adequate preventive interventions. Second, the evaluation of gene expression alterations could be exploited to predict the outcome of treatments and to monitor their *biological* effectiveness in addition to symptomatological assessment.

REFERENCES

Alberts, B., Johnson, A., Lewis, J., Raff, M., Roberts, K., & Walter, P. (2002). *Molecular biology of the cell* (4th ed.). Garland Science.

Belzeaux, R., Lin, R., Ju, C., Chay, M. A., Fiori, L. M., Lutz, P. E., & Turecki, G. (2018). Transcriptomic and epigenomic biomarkers of antidepressant response. *Journal of Affective Disorders*, *233*, 36–44. https://doi.org/10.1016/j.jad.2017.08.087

Berlim, M. T., & Turecki, G. (2007). Definition, assessment, and staging of treatment-resistant refractory major depression: A review of current concepts and methods. *Canadian Journal of Psychiatry/Revue Canadienne de Psychiatrie*, *52*(1), 46–54. http://www.ncbi.nlm.nih.gov/pubmed/17444078

Bustamante, A. C., Aiello, A. E., Galea, S., Ratanatharathorn, A., Noronha, C., Wildman, D. E., & Uddin, M. (2016). Glucocorticoid receptor DNA methylation, childhood maltreatment and major depression. *Journal of Affective Disorders*, *206*, 181–188. https://doi.org/10.1016/j.jad.2016.07.038

Cattane, N., Mora, C., Lopizzo, N., Borsini, A., Maj, C., Pedrini, L., & Cattaneo, A. (2019). Identification of a miRNAs signature associated with exposure to stress early in life and enhanced vulnerability for schizophrenia: New insights for the key role of miR-125b-1-3p in neurodevelopmental processes. *Schizophrenia Research*, *205*, 63–75. https://doi.org/10.1016/j.schres.2018.07.030

Cattaneo, A., Cattane, N., Malpighi, C., Czamara, D., Suarez, A., Mariani, N., & Pariante, C. M. (2018). FoxO1, A2M, and TGF-β1: Three novel genes predicting depression in gene X environment interactions are identified using cross-species and cross-tissues transcriptomic and miRNomic analyses. *Molecular Psychiatry*, *23*(11), 2192–2208. https://doi.org/10.1038/s41380-017-0002-4

Ciobanu, L. G., Sachdev, P. S., Trollor, J. N., Reppermund, S., Thalamuthu, A., Mather, K. A., & Baune, B. T. (2016). Differential gene expression in brain and peripheral tissues in depression across the life span: A review of replicated findings. *Neuroscience and Biobehavioral Reviews*, *71*, 281–293. https://doi.org/10.1016/j.neubiorev.2016.08.018

Danese, A., & van Harmelen, A. L. (2017). The hidden wounds of childhood trauma. *European Journal of Psychotraumatology*, *8*(Supp 3), 1375840. https://doi.org/10.1080/20008198.2017.1375840

Dias de Mattos Souza, L., Lopez Molina, M., Azevedo da Silva, R., & Jansen, K. (2016). History of childhood trauma as risk factors to suicide risk in major depression. *Psychiatry Research*, *246*, 612–616. https://doi.org/10.1016/j.psychres.2016.11.002

Ferrúa, C. P., Giorgi, R., da Rosa, L. C., do Amaral, C. C., Ghisleni, G. C., Pinheiro, R. T., & Nedel, F. (2019). MicroRNAs expressed in depression and their associated pathways: A systematic review and a bioinformatics analysis. *Journal of Chemical Neuroanatomy*, *100*, 101650. https://doi.org/10.1016/j.jchemneu.2019.101650

Gabilondo, A., Rojas-Farreras, S., Vilagut, G., Haro, J. M., Fernández, A., Pinto-Meza, A., & Alonso, J. (2010). Epidemiology of major depressive episode in a southern European country: Results from the ESEMeD-Spain project. *Journal of Affective Disorders*, *120*(1–3), 76–85. https://doi.org/10.1016/j.jad.2009.04.016

Gaudiano, B. A., & Zimmerman, M. (2010). The relationship between childhood trauma history and the psychotic subtype of major depression. *Acta Psychiatrica Scandinavica*, *121*(6), 462–470. https://doi.org/10.1111/j.1600-0447.2009.01477.x

Hasin, D. S., Sarvet, A. L., Meyers, J. L., Saha, T. D., Ruan, W. J., Stohl, M., & Grant, B. F. (2018). Epidemiology of adult DSM-5 major depressive disorder and its specifiers in the United States. *JAMA Psychiatry*, *75*(4), 336–346. https://doi.org/10.1001/jamapsychiatry.2017.4602

Infurna, M. R., Reichl, C., Parzer, P., Schimmenti, A., Bifulco, A., & Kaess, M. (2016). Associations between depression and specific childhood experiences of abuse and neglect: A meta-analysis. *Journal of Affective Disorders, 190,* 47–55. https://doi.org/10.1016/j.jad.2015.09.006

Jansen, R., Penninx, B. W. J. H., Madar, V., Xia, K., Milaneschi, Y., Hottenga, J. J., & Sullivan, P. F. (2016). Gene expression in major depressive disorder. *Molecular Psychiatry, 21*(3), 339–347. https://doi.org/10.1038/mp.2015.57

Kautzky, A., Dold, M., Bartova, L., Spies, M., Kranz, G. S., Souery, D., & Kasper, S. (2019). Clinical factors predicting treatment resistant depression: Affirmative results from the European multicenter study. *Acta Psychiatrica Scandinavica, 139*(1), 78–88. https://doi.org/10.1111/acps.12959

Kéri, S., Szabó, C., & Kelemen, O. (2014). Blood biomarkers of depression track clinical changes during cognitive-behavioral therapy. *Journal of Affective Disorders, 164,* 118–122. https://doi.org/10.1016/j.jad.2014.04.030

Kolshus, E., Ryan, K. M., Blackshields, G., Smyth, P., Sheils, O., & McLoughlin, D. M. (2017). Peripheral blood microRNA and VEGFA mRNA changes following electroconvulsive therapy: Implications for psychotic depression. *Acta Psychiatrica Scandinavica, 136*(6), 594–606. https://doi.org/10.1111/acps.12821

Labonté, B., Suderman, M., Maussion, G., Navaro, L., Yerko, V., Mahar, I., & Turecki, G. (2012). Genome-wide epigenetic regulation by early-life trauma. *Archives of General Psychiatry, 69*(7), 722–731. https://doi.org/10.1001/archgenpsychiatry.2011.2287

Mandelli, L., Petrelli, C., & Serretti, A. (2015). The role of specific early trauma in adult depression: A meta-analysis of published literature. Childhood Trauma and Adult Depression. *European Psychiatry: The Journal of the Association of European Psychiatrists, 30*(6), 665–680. https://doi.org/10.1016/j.eurpsy.2015.04.007

McGowan, P. O., & Matthews, S. G. (2018). Prenatal stress, glucocorticoids, and developmental programming of the stress response. *Endocrinology, 159*(1), 69–82. https://doi.org/10.1210/en.2017-00896

McGowan, P. O., & Szyf, M. (2010). The epigenetics of social adversity in early life: Implications for mental health outcomes. *Neurobiology of Disease, 39*(1), 66–72. https://doi.org/10.1016/j.nbd.2009.12.026

Minelli, A., Magri, C., Giacopuzzi, E., & Gennarelli, M. (2018). The effect of childhood trauma on blood transcriptome expression in major depressive disorder. *Journal of Psychiatric Research, 104,* 50–54. https://doi.org/10.1016/j.jpsychires.2018.06.014

Minelli, A., Zampieri, E., Sacco, C., Bazzanella, R., Mezzetti, N., Tessari, E., & Bortolomasi, M. (2019). Clinical efficacy of trauma-focused psychotherapies in treatment-resistant depression (TRD) in-patients: A randomized, controlled pilot-study. *Psychiatry Research, 273,* 567–574. https://doi.org/10.1016/j.psychres.2019.01.070

Negele, A., Kaufhold, J., Kallenbach, L., & Leuzinger-Bohleber, M. (2015). Childhood trauma and its relation to chronic depression in adulthood. *Depression Research and Treatment, 2015,* 650804. https://doi.org/10.1155/2015/650804

Nelson, J., Klumparendt, A., Doebler, P., & Ehring, T. (2017). Childhood maltreatment and characteristics of adult depression: Meta-analysis. *The British Journal of Psychiatry: The Journal of Mental Science, 210*(2), 96–104. https://doi.org/10.1192/bjp.bp.115.180752

Penninx, B. W. J. H., Nolen, W. A., Lamers, F., Zitman, F. G., Smit, J. H., Spinhoven, P., & Beekman, A. T. F. (2011). Two-year course of depressive and anxiety disorders: Results from the Netherlands study of depression and anxiety (NESDA). *Journal of Affective Disorders, 133*(1–2), 76–85. https://doi.org/10.1016/j.jad.2011.03.027

Poole, J. C., Dobson, K. S., & Pusch, D. (2017). Childhood adversity and adult depression: The protective role of psychological resilience. *Child Abuse & Neglect, 64,* 89–100. https://doi.org/10.1016/j.chiabu.2016.12.012

Spindola, L. M., Pan, P. M., Moretti, P. N., Ota, V. K., Santoro, M. L., Cogo-Moreira, H., & Belangero, S. I. (2017). Gene expression in blood of children and adolescents: Mediation between childhood maltreatment and major depressive disorder. *Journal of Psychiatric Research, 92*, 24–30. https://doi.org/10.1016/j.jpsychires.2017.03.015

Suderman, M., Borghol, N., Pappas, J. J., Pinto Pereira, S. M., Pembrey, M., Hertzman, C., & Szyf, M. (2014). Childhood abuse is associated with methylation of multiple loci in adult DNA. *BMC Medical Genomics, 7*, Article 13. https://doi.org/10.1186/1755-8794-7-13

Thomas, L., Kessler, D., Campbell, J., Morrison, J., Peters, T. J., Williams, C., & Wiles, N. (2013). Prevalence of treatment-resistant depression in primary care: Cross-sectional data. *The British Journal of General Practice: The Journal of the Royal College of General Practitioners, 63*(617), e852–e858. https://doi.org/10.3399/bjgp13X675430

Trivedi, M. H., Rush, A. J., Wisniewski, S. R., Nierenberg, A. A., Warden, D., Ritz, L., & STAR*D Study Team. (2006). Evaluation of outcomes with citalopram for depression using measurement-based care in STAR*D: Implications for clinical practice. *The American Journal of Psychiatry, 163*(1), 28–40. https://doi.org/10.1176/appi.ajp.163.1.28

Tunnard, C., Rane, L. J., Wooderson, S. C., Markopoulou, K., Poon, L., Fekadu, A., & Cleare, A. J. (2014). The impact of childhood adversity on suicidality and clinical course in treatment-resistant depression. *Journal of Affective Disorders, 152-154*, 122–130. https://doi.org/10.1016/j.jad.2013.06.037

Volk, N., Pape, J. C., Engel, M., Zannas, A. S., Cattane, N., Cattaneo, A., & Chen, A. (2016). Amygdalar MicroRNA-15a is essential for coping with chronic stress. *Cell Reports, 17*(7), 1882–1891. https://doi.org/10.1016/j.celrep.2016.10.038

Watkeys, O. J., Kremerskothen, K., Quidé, Y., Fullerton, J. M., & Green, M. J. (2018). Glucocorticoid receptor gene (*NR3C1*) DNA methylation in association with trauma, psychopathology, transcript expression, or genotypic variation: A systematic review. *Neuroscience and Biobehavioral Reviews, 95*, 85–122. https://doi.org/10.1016/j.neubiorev.2018.08.017

Williams, L. M., Debattista, C., Duchemin, A. M., Schatzberg, A. F., & Nemeroff, C. B. (2016). Childhood trauma predicts antidepressant response in adults with major depression: Data from the randomized international study to predict optimized treatment for depression. *Translational Psychiatry, 6*(5), e799. https://doi.org/10.1038/tp.2016.61

12

Consequences for Practical Work With EMDR Therapy

Arne Hofmann and Marilyn Luber

INTRODUCTION

In this chapter, we discuss some practical consequences of the paradigm shift to understand depression as a stress- and trauma-based disorder. As successful eye movement desensitization and reprocessing (EMDR) therapy helps to resolve stress- and trauma-based memories, the authors show how EMDR therapy works with depressive patients. Randomized controlled trial (RCT) studies demonstrate that not only is EMDR therapy for depressive disorders at least equal to other treatments, but there are more complete remissions. The EMDR DeprEnd Protocol is a significant step forward in the treatment of depressive patients and in the reduction of depressive relapses. This is important as the effect of treatment-resistant depression leaves patients at risk for suicide and families to bear the loss of their family member. Improved treatment possibilities would also occasion economic savings. With more knowledge about the importance of childhood memories in development of depression, we can also do much more for primary prevention of depression.

THE IMPORTANCE OF ADVERSE LIFE EXPERIENCES AND PATHOGENIC MEMORIES

A growing number of researchers and clinical practitioners who deal with depressive patients have recently come to the conclusion that distressing and traumatic life experiences play a central role in the development of depressive disorders. This means that depression can be considered a trauma- and stressor-related disorder.

From the perspective of the illness model in EMDR therapy and our clinical experience, distressing and traumatic life events and the pathological memories resulting from them are crucial factors in the development and perseverance of depressive episodes. Pathogenic memories are biologically active with cognitive and affective consequences lasting long after the distressing experience was triggered. They respond only to a limited extent to talk psychotherapy (Centonze et al., 2005; Hase et al., 2017). After successful EMDR therapy, both pathogenic memories and the symptoms that arise because of them resolve well. This suggests that using a therapy that is very effective for traumatized patients, such as EMDR therapy, will be effective in the treatment of depressive patients as well. In this book, the authors report on their experience of more than a decade of successfully implementing EMDR therapy with depressive patients in order to process pathogenic memories.

EMDR THERAPY AND RANDOMIZED CONTROLLED TRIALS

In a number of RCT studies, it was shown that using EMDR therapy for depressive disorders is at least equivalent in comparison to the treatments used to date, but also achieves considerably more complete remissions. In a number of cases and case series, this appears to lead to a more significant improvement than would generally be expected and to the complete disappearance of depressive relapses. If this finding could be further solidified through scientific research, it would have wide-reaching consequences for the lives of millions of depressed people, their ability to work, their close social relationships, and their ability to raise their children with good emotional contact. Additionally, thousands of relatives would be spared the fate of a family made smaller by suicide, and economically, a larger number of resources could be made available for other purposes.

At the time of this book's completion, however, there are still no sufficiently large controlled studies with long enough follow ups that would ultimately prove scientifically that EMDR is better in preventing depressive relapses than other psychotherapy approaches. In our opinion, a study of this kind is crucial. But even without it, there are already important consequences that can be drawn from the available study results we have so far and from our experience.

CONSEQUENCES FOR THE TREATMENT OF DEPRESSIVE DISORDERS

During history taking for depressive patients, any distressing life experiences as well as comorbidities with trauma- and stressor-related disorders should be obtained. This is especially the case when distressing life experiences have a temporal connection with the beginning of the depressive episode and applies particularly to recurrent or chronic depression as well as depressive disorders that have not sufficiently responded to previous treatments. Here, EMDR therapy should be considered as an important treatment option.

In the treatment of depressive disorders with EMDR, the Episode Triggers, belief systems, and also Suicidal and Depressive States, which in some cases become a stand-alone problem, are brought into focus and processed with EMDR. The practical steps of diagnosis and treatment were described in the preceding book chapters in detail. When a present depressive episode has abated, additional pathogenic memories are also processed with EMDR as a form of relapse prevention (e.g., distressing and traumatic life experiences from childhood and adolescence). By processing these earlier memories as well, the risk for another depressive episode appears to reduce considerably.

A particular clinical problem is presented by depressive patients with severe comorbidities, particularly those with a severe trauma- and stressor-related disorder. These are often not sufficiently diagnosed in clinical practice and necessitate a longer and more complex treatment than other depressive patients. This must be taken into consideration when working with these patients.

CONSEQUENCES FOR RESEARCH

In light of the current availability of nine RCTs demonstrating the success of EMDR therapy in treating depression, further research into EMDR therapy to treat different kinds of depression is strongly recommended.

Due to the economic savings that would be possible with improved treatment options—particularly for recurrent and chronic depression—public funding should be sought, for example, through cooperation with insurance companies responsible for a large part of the costs for these patients.

It would be particularly important in the future to have larger treatment studies with different populations suffering from depression and particularly the investigation of long-term outcomes with question of the long-lasting consequences of treatment.

CONSEQUENCES FOR PRIMARY PREVENTION AND THE PROTECTION OF CHILDREN

There is a broad consensus among researchers that distressing and traumatic experiences in childhood play a decisive role in many cases of depression in the form of risk factors, triggers, and also complicating factors in treatment.

In light of the frequency of depressive disorders, considerably more attention must be devoted to the known primary causes. The known primary consequences include physical, sexual, and verbal violence, as well as neglect. Precisely in these four areas, children still remain—to a great extent—unprotected against violence and neglect. Some researchers in Germany have described this situation as an epidemic. In larger epidemiological studies, it is shown that traumatic experiences and the experience of a dysfunctional home situation in childhood appear to be responsible for a large portion of the risk for major depression and suicide (Dube et al., 2001, 2003).

Even if increasing activity can be documented on the topic of child protection in recent years, there has been little improvement to stop the continuation of the mechanisms of harm by families with, for example, mentally ill parents as well as single parents and groups of offenders. This urgently needs to be improved. All of these items are only partial contributions to the solution of a problem that is complex. Changing these contributors to depression certainly would help make an increasing number of depressive disorders, that in the future will otherwise be predictable, easier to treat and increasingly improve the primary prevention of depressive disorders long-term, for example, through more robust child protection.

REFERENCES

Centonze, D., Siracusano, A., Calabresi, P., & Bernardi, G. (2005). Removing pathogenic memories: A neurobiology of psychotherapy. *Molecular Psychiatry, 32*(2), 123–132. https://doi.org/10.1385/MN:32:2:123

Dube, S. R., Anda, R. F., Felitti, V. J., Chapman, D. P., Williamson, D. F., & Giles, W. H. (2001). Childhood abuse, household dysfunction, and the risk of attempted suicide throughout the life span: Findings from the Adverse Childhood Experiences Study. *JAMA, 286*(24), 3089–3096. https://doi.org/10.1001/jama.286.24.3089

Dube, S. R., Felitti, V., Dong, M., Chapman, D. P., Giles, W. H., & Anda, R. (2003). Childhood abuse, neglect, and household dysfunction and the risk of illicit drug use: The adverse childhood experiences study. *Pediatrics, 111*(3), 564–572. https://doi.org/10.1542/peds.111.3.564

Hase, M., Balmaceda, U. M., Ostacoli, L., Liebermann, P., & Hofmann, A. (2017). The AIP Model of EMDR therapy and pathogenic memories. *Frontiers in Psychology, 8*, Article 1578. https://doi.org/10.3389/fpsyg.2017.01578

Resources

IV

13

Randomized Controlled Scientific Studies on EMDR and Depression

Sara Carletto, Francesca Malandrone, and Luca Ostacoli

TABLE 13.1. Randomized Controlled Scientific Studies on EMDR and Depression

NR	AUTHOR/YEAR	N	INTERVENTION	DIAGNOSIS	INSTRUMENTS	RESULTS
1	Dominguez et al. (2020)	49	CBT with additional 3 sessions EMDR versus AT versus TAU	MD in psychiatric outpatients	DASS-42	After EMDR significantly fewer MD versus AT and TAU, at 6 and 12 weeks follow-up
2	Minelli et al. (2019)	22	24 sessions EMDR or TF-CBT	Treatment-resistant depression	BDI-II, MADRS	Significant improvement after EMDR and TF-CBT. Improvements only stable in EMDR group after 3 months
3	Fereidouni et al. (2019)	70	9 sessions EMDR versus TAU	Major depression with suicidal thoughts	BSSI	Significantly higher reduction of suicidal thoughts after EMDR
4	Ostacoli et al. (2018)	66	15 +/- 3 sessions EMDR or CBT	Recurrent depression in psychiatric outpatients	BDI-II, MINI	Similar improvement in both conditions. At treatment's end, BDI-II significantly better in EMDR group
5	Hase et al. (2018)	30	4–12 sessions EMDR versus TAU	Inpatients with depression	BDI-II, SCL-90-R	50% remission in EMDR + TAU versus 25% in TAU alone. EMDR results stable after 1 year
6	Su et al. (2018)**	12+8	Part 1: 12 patients had 10 sessions EMDR. Part 2: 8 patients had 4 sessions CBT versus EMDR	Depressive outpatients	PHQ-9, MINI	Part 1: 10 of 12 reported improvement or remission. Part 2: EMDR and CBT both similar and effective

Chapter 13 Scientific Studies on EMDR and Depression

#	Study	N	Intervention	Population	Measures	Results
7	Gauhar (2016)	26	6–8 EMDR sessions versus WL	Depressive patients without ADM	BDI-II, SCL-90, QoL	Significant improvement in EMDR versus WL. After 3 months stable
8	Mogahadam et al. (2015)	60	3 sessions EMDR versus TAU	Patients with depression after myocardial infarction	BDI-II	Significant reduction in EMDR versus TAU (BDI <17). Results stable after 12 months
9	Hogan (2001)*	38	4 sessions CBT + EMDR versus 4 CBT sessions	Depression, dysthymia, or adjustment disorder with depressive symptoms	BDI-II, SCL-90-R, SIS	All treatments similarly effective. In 4 EMDR patients, speedy, almost full remission (not in CBT)

*Dissertation.
**Master's thesis.

ADM, antidepressant medication; AT, assertiveness training; BDI, Beck Depression Inventory; BDI-II, Beck Depression Inventory, Second Edition; BSSI, Beck Scale for Suicidal Ideation; CBT, cognitive behavioral therapy; DASS-42, Depression, Anxiety, and Stress Scale; EMDR, eye movement desensitization and reprocessing; MADRS, Montgomery–Åsberg Depression Rating Scale; MD, major depression; MINI, Mini International Neuropsychiatric Interview; PHQ-9, Patient Health Questionnaire–9 (part of DSM-IV); QoL, quality of life; SCL-90, Symptom Checklist-90; SCL-90-R, Symptom Checklist-90-Revised; SIS, Session Impact Scale; TAU, treatment as usual; TF-CBT, trauma-focused cognitive behavioral therapy; WL, waiting list.

Source: Updated by Dr. Arne Hofmann and derived from Malandrone, F., Carletto, S., Hase, M., Hofmann, A., & Ostacoli, L. (2019). A brief narrative summary of randomized controlled trials investigating EMDR treatment of patients with depression. *Journal of EMDR Practice and Research*, 13(4), 302–306. https://doi.org/10.1891/1933-3196.13.4.302

14

How to Fill the Symptom Event Map

Arne Hofmann

The Symptom Event Map is one of the most important tools for treatment planning in the DeprEnd Protocol for the treatment of depression as it charts depressive episodes and their intensity, Episode Triggers, and Compensation Zones. The processing of Episode Triggers often helps significantly to relieve the symptoms of depressive episodes. The Symptom Event Map is made up of two unrelated maps that, if pulled together, allow for the identification of the events that triggered specific depressive episodes to be clearly pictured and later used as targets in eye movement desensitization and reprocessing (EMDR) therapy. What is different in this map is that because there are two maps put together, there are two "x" axes turned on their sides and inhabiting the space of the "y" axis.

The first of the two maps is the *symptom map*. This map is plotted in an unusual way with the x-axis situated on the right side of the Symptom Event Map. On this map, depressive episodes, major depression, and dysthymia, as well as manic episodes, can be documented. In classic psychiatric literature, a depressive episode is drawn as a dip in the baseline that is the continuous dotted line of well-being on the map a little above the middle of the map ("no depression" is labelled on the right x-axis). If the patient gets more depressed, the line can drop from the baseline to the level of Medium Depression or even to Severe Depression. Likewise, but often not written on the map, manic or hypomanic episodes could be documented with the line drawn above the level of the baseline.

When the symptom line goes back to baseline after a depressive dip, this indicates that the patient was able to recover fully after this particular depressive episode. If this happens, it is of great importance, as it indicates a phase called the *Compensation Zone*. In most cases, this event signals that the depressive episodes and Episode Triggers that occur before this Compensation Zone are not primary targets for EMDR in the first phase of treatment.

If the patient becomes dysthymic, the symptom line dips below the baseline.

Note: The timeline on the bottom of the map has no ages charted; this is so it can be adjusted to the age of a specific patient. Also, it is not necessary to document the full age range of the patient; it is more important to focus on the depressive episodes and Episode Triggers that are needed for treatment planning.

The unrelated second map is a *trauma map*, which is located on the left x-axis. The beginning of the scale indicates no stressful/distressing events or 0, while the top shows the most stressful events or 10. The stressful life events, including or not including Criterion A, are indicated on the horizontal line labelled "Years" and then the event itself appears at the appropriate Subjective Units of Distress (SUD) level with a dot.

When the two maps are blended together, the stressful life events give a clear picture of their time relative to the beginning of the depressive episodes and can also identify and show the Episode Triggers. The Episode Triggers usually have a high SUD and occur 1 or 2 months before the depressive episode begins. With this map, the most important memories that EMDR therapy needs to process in depressive patients can clearly be identified in most cases: they are the Episode Triggers.

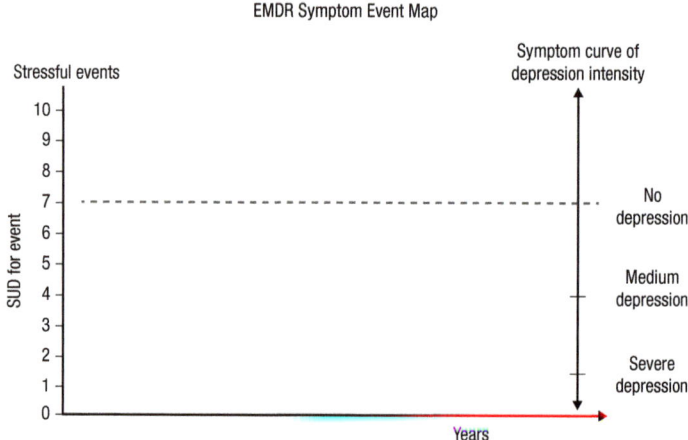

FIGURE 14.1. The empty Symptom Event Map: On the timeline, when drawing the first map, the strength of symptoms is given as a curve (right-side scale/Symptom Curve). Connected with this is the second map (on the left-side scale) with the distressing memories that are recorded with their SUDs on the timeline. Both maps are different, but the combination allows the identification of depressive Episode Triggers.

EMDR, eye movement desensitization and reprocessing; SUD, Subjective Units of Distress.

Here are the steps to use the Symptom Event Map:

1. *List Depressive Episodes:* Make a list of the depressive episodes of the patient (if the list is very long, the current and worst are most important).
2. *Find the Compensation Zones:* Find out the times a patient felt good and was not depressed between the trauma or depressive episodes; these are the Compensation Zones.
3. *Chart the Depressive Episodes:* Begin the map on the left side with either the last Compensation Zone or with the first depressive episode (the dotted line at "no depression" belongs only to the right-side scale).
4. *Indicate Depression Intensity:* Draw the symptom curve that describes the intensity of the feeling of being depressed as a dip in the line on the map (looking at the right-side of the scale for the depression intensity—from hypomanic to No Depression to Severe Depression).

5. *Plot Stressful Events on Chart at SUDs Level:* Plot the list of stressful life events—including attachment-related traumatic and Criterion A events—that occurred during that time along the horizontal line labelled "Years" and write down their SUDs. The stressful events (other than the depressive episodes that are shown as dips from the baseline) are written as dots on the map.
6. *Plot Dots and Their SUDs on Map:* Put the dots of these events on the map with their SUDs and where they occur related to the chronological age.
7. *Identify Episode Triggers:* Look 2 months before the beginning of the depressive episodes and you usually can identify the Episode Triggers (in most cases, losses, separations, and humiliations).
8. *Use the Symptom Event Map as a Therapy Planning Tool:* These Episode Triggers are a *key* element of our treatment that trigger and maintain the depressive episodes and are usually the first targets reprocessed with EMDR.

Here is an example case of how to fill the Symptom Event Map:

This case concerns a 55-year-old manager who is suffering from a severe depressive episode beginning 5 months ago. These are the eight steps used to fill in this Symptom Event Map. Note the dotted line that indicates "No Depression"; this indicates the patient's baseline.

1. *List Depressive Episodes:* The map begins on the left side (as in most cases) in a phase of well-being on the dotted line shortly before the first depressive episode that occurred 5 years before the patient came in for treatment; there is a dip from the baseline to the point on the map that indicates a Medium Depression, and it is labelled "1." on the map in Figure 14.2. A second depressive episode occurred 5 months before the patient came for treatment. The symptom line dips down from the baseline to indicate that this is a Severe Depression and is labelled "2." in Figure 14.2 and is why the patient came into treatment. After the prior/first depressive episode, the patient had recovered fully from it without any therapy. The stressful events (other than the depressive episodes that are shown as dips from the baseline) are written as dots on the map.
2. *Find the Compensation Zones:* The time between the end of the first episode and the beginning of the current episode can be seen as a complete remission of depressive symptoms and a Compensation Zone.
3. *Chart the Last Compensation Zone or First Depressive Event:* Both depressive episodes are drawn on the symptom line of the map (following the axis on the right side). The space between the episodes on the well-being line is the Compensation Zone. For this patient, his Compensation Zone was from about 51 to 55 years of age.
4. *Indicate Depression Intensity:* In Figure 14.2, "1." indicates the dip of the earlier episode (Medium); "2." indicates the dip of the second depressive episode (Severe).
5. *Plot Stressful Events on Chart at SUDs Level:* There are two critical events (the dots on the map) that have a time relationship with the depressive episodes, which are indicated on the map by dips down from the baseline.
6. *Plot Dots and Their SUDs on Map:* The dots on the map indicate two events that occurred shortly before the depressive episodes began: bullying before the medium depressive episode and the death of his wife before the severe depressive episode.

7. *Identify Episode Triggers:* There are two Episode Triggers. Four weeks before the current depressive episode, the patient's wife died. The patient gave the memory of the event a SUD of 9/10 (marked "4." on the map in Figure 14.2). Five years before, when the first depressive episode occurred, there was an Episode Trigger 2 months before the beginning of the prior depressive episode. At that time, the patient was laid off from his job after a period of bullying (marked "3." on the map in Figure 14.2). The SUDs for the events are shown on the left side of the map where the SUDs are indicated.
8. *Use the Symptom Event Map as a Therapy Planning Tool:* The Symptom Event Map in Figure 14.2 gives therapists a planning tool for targeting and sequencing the stressful life events that occurred before the depressive episodes. Usually, we begin by targeting the trigger of the current episode (indicated as point "4." in Figure 14.2) to relieve the symptoms of the current episode. In this case, with the loss of a partner, the SUD probably will not go down to zero and the patient will still be in mourning after the processing of the memories of the death of the partner. Nevertheless, most patients have a significant reduction of their current depressive symptoms after processing the related Episode Trigger. In the best case, the patient can, after the event is processed with EMDR, move back into the Compensation Zone achieved before the partner's death.

Even if patients reach a full remission after the reprocessing of the Episode Trigger of the current episode, it is recommended to look for other significant stressful memories and reprocess them, even if they do not cause symptoms currently. This is important for *relapse prevention*. This probably would be the case for the Episode Trigger of the earlier and first episode (indicated as point "3." in Figure 14.2).

The processing of Episode Triggers is one of the key instruments to treat depressive episodes, but, in some cases, this is not enough. In these cases, we look for the other targets described in this book, such as negative belief systems and Depressive or Suicidal States.

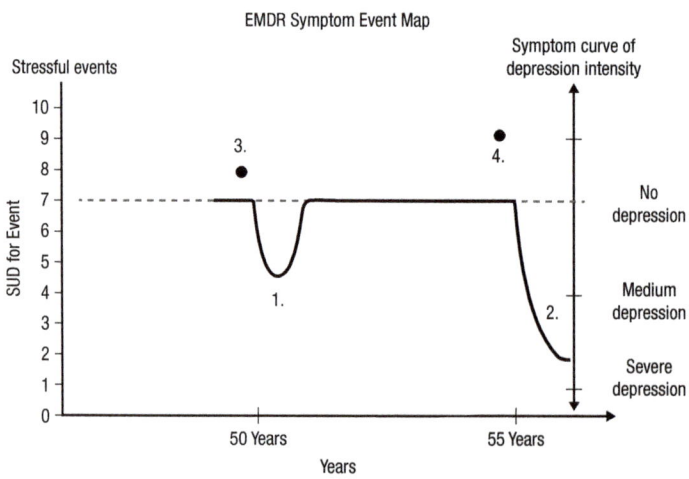

FIGURE 14.2. The filled Symptom Event Map of the 55-year-old patient.

EMDR, eye movement desensitization and reprocessing; SUD, Subjective Units of Distress.

15

Finding a Certified EMDR Therapist

Marilyn Luber and Arne Hofmann

Don't worry; many people suffering from depressive symptoms respond well to the established treatments for depression recommended in current scientific guidelines. If this is the case, additional eye movement desensitization and reprocessing (EMDR) treatment may not be necessary. In addition, there are a number of depressive disorders that do not have primarily psychological causes, but rather organic causes (hormonal changes, side effects of medications, etc.). In order not to overlook these forms of depressive disorders, it is important to involve the primary care physician or psychiatric specialist in the treatment of depressive disorders.

A different situation exists when depressive relapses occur repeatedly (recurrent depression) or a depressive episode does not resolve, even with treatment, or does not respond satisfactorily to treatment. This is especially the case when traumatic or other severe, stressful experiences (especially losses, separations, shaming or humiliation) have occurred to the affected person and the memories of these are still stressful in the present. In such a situation, EMDR therapy can be very helpful.

The current scientific status of research on EMDR therapy for depressive disorders is still evolving and recognition of EMDR treatment must be also taken into account. EMDR therapy is recognized internationally in the guidelines for treating posttraumatic stress disorder (PTSD). Even though there are currently nine randomized controlled trials (RCTs) in the area of treatment of depression that show that EMDR therapy is successful and at least equivalent to conventional psychotherapy treatments, there is still no recognition for EMDR therapy for depression in international guidelines. These recognition processes currently need to have more data such as more studies and time. The studies are evolving as a result of the work of the authors in this book and by others in the field.

In EMDR treatment, there is a clear relationship between the effectiveness of the EMDR treatment and the qualification of the treating therapists. First and foremost, this includes the basic professional qualification of the therapist, that is, the license to practice as a psychotherapist. Furthermore, it is essential to establish the quality of the therapist's EMDR training.

EMDR is unfortunately not a trademarked term, so *EMDR* may now be used by a wide range of professionals who have not been trained formally (or at all) or are trained by therapists who are not qualified themselves. Patients need to be well-informed about how to select an EMDR-certified clinician to make sure that they receive the type of EMDR therapy treatment that is needed.

It is therefore important to check that the EMDR provider being considered for treatment is appropriately qualified to deliver EMDR therapy and has some experience in treating depressive disorders with EMDR. Ask if the provider has experience working with depressive disorders and trauma.

The international professional societies for EMDR have lists of EMDR-certified therapists on their websites:

- EMDR International Association (EMDRIA) for the United States: www.emdria.org
- EMDR Canada: www.emdrcanada.org
- EMDR European Association: www.emdr-europe.org
- EMDR Asia: www.emdrasia.org

When looking for a good EMDR therapist, as with all psychotherapeutic treatments, the basic feeling during the first trial sessions is still crucial. This basic feeling, the *positive chemistry* with the therapist, is one of the most important factors in predicting a positive treatment outcome. If there is this positive feeling in the therapeutic relationship and the therapist is appropriately qualified in the EMDR field, the chances for successful EMDR therapy are very good.

Index

ACEs. *See* adverse childhood experiences
active depression, 47
Adaptive Information Processing (AIP) Model, 11, 23–27, 32, 42, 46, 100–102, 111, 122–123, 130, 132
adverse childhood experiences (ACEs), 9–10, 138
adverse life experiences, 195–196
affective spectrum, 172
affects, 28
AIP Model. *See* Adaptive Information Processing Model
alternating visual bilateral stimulation (AVBS), 176
anabolism, 62
anger, 55
antidepressants, 5–6, 121–122, 184
anxiety disorders, 32
attachment adversity, 185
Attachment Cry, 59
attachment trauma, 9
autonomic nervous system, 58–63
autonomic regulation, 62
AVBS. *See* alternating visual bilateral stimulation

BDNF. *See* brain-derived neurotrophic factor
Beck, Aaron, 110
belief systems treatment with EMDR therapy, 109–119
   depressive episode with somatic symptoms, case study, 110
   memory network, 112–117
   negative belief systems, 109–117
      case studies, 112–119
      and depressive patients, 111–117
      history, 110–111
      processing, 109–117
   triggers, working with, 117–118
benzodiazepines, 184
bipolar disorders, 4
   brain-derived neurotrophic factor, 173–174
   case study, 178
   etiology of, 173–174
   treatment of, 174–177
      EMDR for, 175–177
      practical experience, 177
      stabilization techniques for, 177
bipolar I disorder, 172–173
bipolar II disorder, 172–173
body screening of polyvagal state, 63–67
brain-derived neurotrophic factor (BDNF), 173–174
bullying, 9

candidate genes, 8
Caspi, Avshalom, 8
CBT. *See* cognitive behavioral therapy
certified EMDR therapists, 209–210
childhood attachment traumas, 9
childhood trauma, 184–185
children, protection of, 197
chronic depression, 47
chronic psychosocial stress at work, 9
cognitive behavioral therapy (CBT), 7, 110
comorbidity with complex trauma-related disorders, EMDR therapy and, 137–144
   case studies, 139–143
   C-PTSD, 138–141
   depression, 138–144
   dissociative depression, 141–144
   understanding of, 137–138
Compensation Zone, 103
complex posttraumatic stress disorder (C-PTSD), 97–99, 137–141
   EMDR-DI Protocol for, 145–166

corticotropin-releasing factor (CRF), 187
C-PTSD. *See* complex posttraumatic stress disorder
CRF. *See* corticotropin-releasing factor
cyclothymia, 172

default mode network (DMN), 176
DeprEnd Protocol, EMDR therapy, 39–51
  clinical experience and example cases, 48–51
  Depressive and Suicidal States, processing of, 46
  Episode Triggers, processing of, 44–45
  future work for Episode Triggers, 45
  history taking, 42–44
  negative belief systems, processing of, 45
  overview, 41–42
  preparation and stabilization, 44, 53–89
  relapse prevention, 46, 129–136
  scientific background, 39–41
  strategies for structuring reprocessing according to clinical situation, 46–51
  triggers in, 45, 131
depressed mood, 53, 121
depression, 1–14, 26, 32–33, 138–144
  active, 47
  Beck's view of, 110
  causes of, 53–54
  childhood trauma and, 184–185
  chronic, 47, 184–185
  clinical presentations of, 99–107
    chronic depression with/without adverse childhood experience/complex post-traumatic stress disorder, 106–107
    double depression with/without adverse childhood experience/complex post-traumatic stress disorder, 105–106
    recurrent depressive episodes, 102–103
    recurrent episodes with adverse childhood experience complex posttraumatic stress disorder, 103–105
    single depressive episode, 100–102
  and dissociative depression, 141–144
  emotions
    psychoeducation for, 55–57
    regulating volume of, 57–58
  exclusion criteria, 54
  features, 53–54
  ICD-10 characterization of, 3–4, 53–54
  largely in remission, 47
  stressful life events and, 184–185
  tolerance, window of, 58–63
depressive antecedents, 5

depressive disorders, 3–5
  antidepressive medications for, 5
  attachment trauma and, 9
  causes, 7–11
  experiences, 2, 5, 7–13
  genetic factors, 8
  ICD-10 characterization of, 3–4, 53–54
  incidence of, 4
  medications for treatment of, 6–7
  pathogenic memories and, 11–12
  possibilities for treatment and their limits, 5–7
  psychopharmacological interventions for, 7
  risk factors, 4–5
  stressors, 9
  suicide and, 4
  therapeutic approaches for treatment of, 6–7
  treatment with EMDR therapy
    AIP Model, 24–25
    consequences for, 196–197
    DeprEnd Protocol, 39–51
    eight phases of, 27–29
    first systematic investigations, 12–14
    history of, 1–3, 23–24
    mechanism of action of, 29–32
    in mouse experiment, 30
    overview, 23
    pathogenic memories and, 11–12, 25–27
    resources in, 27
    variability, 5
depressive episodes, 4–5
  recurrent, 102–103
  single, 100–102
  with somatic symptoms, 110
depressive relapses, 6
Depressive/Suicidal States, with EMDR therapy, 121–126
  body memories of, 121–122
  clinical experiences and example cases, 123–126
  clinical indications of, 122–123
  memories of being, 122–123
diaphragmatic breathing, 58, 68–69
diet, risk factor for depression, 86–87
disgust, 55
dissociative disorder, 97
DMN. *See* default mode network
double depression, 13

EDEN. *See* European Depression EMDR Network
EEG. *See* electroencephalography
electroencephalography (EEG), 12

Index   213

EMDR therapy. *See* eye movement desensitization and reprocessing (EMDR) therapy
EMDR-DI Protocol. *See* EMDR-Drawing Integration Protocol
EMDR-Drawing Integration (EMDR-DI) Protocol, 145–166
  case study, 158–166
  Depressive States with, 153–154, 158–166
  within desensitization/reprocessing session, 152–153
  goal of, 146
  Self-Contact Technique, 154–157
  technique, 151–152
emotional abuse, 9
emotional scarring, 121–122
emotions
  authentic vs. secondary, 56–57
  enriching, 55–56
  negative, 55
  physical sensations of, 61
  protective, 55–56
  psychoeducation for, 55–57
  regulating volume of, 57–58
    be friendly to ourselves, 57
    container, 57
    diaphragmatic breathing, 58
    emotions are transient and we are greater than they are, 57
    expression, creative, 58
    here and now through the five senses, maintain perception of, 57–58
    movement, 58
    posture, 57
    sharing, 58
  of transformation, 55
enriching emotions, 55–56
Episode Triggers with EMDR therapy, 44–45, 97–107
  definition, 97
  depression, clinical presentations of, 99–107
    chronic depression with or without adverse childhood experience/complex posttraumatic stress disorder, 106–107
    double depression with or without adverse childhood experience/complex posttraumatic stress disorder, 105–106
    recurrent depressive episodes, 102–103
    recurrent episodes with adverse childhood experience complex posttraumatic stress disorder, 103–105
    single depressive episode, 100–102

  distressing life events, processing of, 97–99
  pathogenic memories, clinical manifestation of, 98
    C-PTSD/personality disorder, 98
    depressive disorder triggers, 98
    early childhood memories, 98
  Symptom Event Map and, 97, 205–208
European Depression EMDR Network (EDEN), 13
Everyday Life Test, 27
expression, creative, 58
eye movement desensitization and reprocessing (EMDR) therapy, depressive disorders, 1–3, 12–14, 24–33
  AIP Model of, 24–25
  belief systems treatment, 109–119
  bipolar disorder with, 171–178
  comorbidity with complex trauma-related disorders and, 137–144
  consequences
    for primary prevention, 197
    for protection of children, 197
    for research, 197
    for the treatment, 196–197
  DeprEnd Protocol, 39–51
    clinical experience and example cases, 48–51
    Depressive and Suicidal States, processing of, 46
    Episode Triggers, processing of, 44–45
    history taking, 42–44
    negative belief systems, processing of, 45
    overview, 41–42
    preparation and stabilization, 44, 53–89
    relapse prevention, 46
    scientific background, 39–41
    strategies for structuring reprocessing according to clinical situation, 46–51
    triggers and future work for Episode Triggers, 45
  Depressive/Suicidal States with, 121–126
  eight phases of, 27–29
    assessment phase, 28
    body scan phase, 28
    closure phase, 29
    desensitization phase, 28
    history taking, 27
    installation phase, 28
    patient stabilization, 27–28, 63–67
    reevaluation phase, 29
  Episode Triggers with, 97–107
  history of, 23–24
  mechanism of action of, 29–32

in mouse experiment, 30
pathogenic memories and, 11–12, 25–27
practical work with, 195–197
preparation and stabilization in, 53–89
randomized controlled trials, 196, 202–203
relapse prevention with, 129–136
resources in, 27
eye movements, 29–31

fear, 29–31, 55
fear neurons, 31
felt sense of emotions, 61
fight or flight, 59–63, 66, 155

GABAergic genes, 186
glutamatergic genes, 186
green light, traffic light, 66, 154

habituation, 29
Hakomi's 3-Step Procedure, 71–79
Hamilton Depression Rating Scale, 11, 42, 176
Hidden Heart: The Magic Query, 70–71
History-Taking Test, 28
HPA axis. *See* hypothalamic–pituitary–adrenal axis
Hughes, Karin, 10
human brain, 29–32
hyperactivation, 60
hyperarousal, 59–63
hypoarousal, 59–63
hypomania, 172–173
hypothalamic–pituitary–adrenal (HPA) axis, 86, 187–188

imagery rescripting, 111
immobilization defenses, 59
interpersonal psychotherapy (IPT), 7
interpersonal traumas, 185
IPT. *See* interpersonal psychotherapy

leave and recall technique, 79–85
lifestyle changes, EMDR therapy, 86–88
 diet, 86–87
 physical activity, 86
 sleep, 87
 synergy of EMDR and, 87–88
Likert scale, 12

"magic query," 70–71
major depressive disorder (MDD), 183
 childhood trauma for, 184–185
 chronicity, 183–184
 drug treatment, 184

microRNAs in, 186
molecular mechanisms related to, 185–190
recurrence, 183–184
resistance, 183–184
stressful life events for, 184–185
traumatic events and, 184–190
maladaptive schemata, 111
MDD. *See* major depressive disorder
microRNAs, 186
mirtazapine, 184
mobilization defenses, 59
mood stabilizers, 174, 184
movement, for regulating emotions, 58

NC. *See* negative cognition
negative belief systems treatment with EMDR therapy, 109–117
 case studies, 111–119
 and depressive patients, 111–117
 history, 110–111
 pathogenic memories as cause of, 112
 processing, 109–117
negative cognition (NC), 28
negative emotions, 55

orienting response hypothesis, 29

parasympathetic function, 58–63
pathogenic memories, 11–12, 111, 195–196
PC. *See* positive cognition
peritraumatic dissociation, 47
phonological loop, 29
physical activity, risk factor for depression, 86
physical violence, 9
Polyvagal Theory of Porges, 58, 66
 immobilization defenses, 59
 mobilization defenses, 59
 state of security and affiliation, 58–59
positive cognition (PC), 28
posttraumatic stress disorder (PTSD), 23, 25–26, 32, 47–48, 97, 137–144
posture, for regulating emotions, 57
preparation/stabilization in EMDR therapy for depressive patients, 44, 53–89
 body screening of polyvagal state, 63–67
 depression, core of, 53–63
 diaphragmatic breathing, role of, 68–69
 Hakomi's 3-Step Procedure for, 71–79
 hidden heart, 70–71
 leave and recall technique, 79–85
 lifestyle changes, 86–88
 diet, 86–87
 physical activity, 86

sleep, 87
   synergy of EMDR and, 87–88
   "magic query," 70–71
   Self-Contact Technique, 63–67
   somatic resources, 67–89
   Triple Thanksgiving, 88–89
prolonged grief, 97
protective emotions, 55–56
psychodynamic psychotherapy, 7
psychoeducation
   for emotions, 55–57
   on Self-Contact Technique, 64–67
PTSD. *See* posttraumatic stress disorder

randomized controlled trials (RCTs), 196, 202–203
RCTs. *See* randomized controlled trials
recurrent depressive episodes, 102–103, 184
red light, traffic light, 66, 154
relapse prevention with EMDR therapy, 129–136
   and AIP model, 130–131
   steps
      memory of Depressive States, working with, 135–136
      projections into future, working with, 132–134
      resources, building up, 134–135
      triggers, working with, 131–132
resistance, sympathetic system, 63
rest/digest response, 59–63
Risch, Neil, 8

sadness, 55
Safe Place Test, 27
schema therapy, 111
Self-Contact Technique, 63–67
   instructions for, 65–66
   positions for, 67
   psychoeducational text on, 64–67
   traffic light for, 66, 154
self-healing, 24
sensations, 28
serotonin and norepinephrine reuptake inhibitors (SNRIs), 184
serotonin reuptake inhibitors (SSRIs), 184
serotonin transporter gene, 8
sexual abuse, 9
Shapiro, Francine, 12, 23–24, 131
sharing, for regulating emotions, 58
simulated death, 60
single depressive episode, 100–102
sleep disturbances, relationship to depression, 87

SNRIs. *See* serotonin and norepinephrine reuptake inhibitors
somatic resources, 67–89
   alignment, 69
   grounding, 69
   hidden heart, 70–71
   leave and recall technique, 79–85
   magic query, 70–71
   memories of, 71–79
SSRIs. *See* serotonin reuptake inhibitors
stabilization in EMDR therapy for depressive disorders, 53–89
   Self-Contact Technique, 63–67
      instructions for, 65–66
      psychoeducational text on, 64–67
   state of security and affiliation, 58–59
Stimulation Test, 28
stressful life events, 184–185
stressors, 9
Subjective Units of Disturbance (SUD), 12, 28
SUD. *See* Subjective Units of Disturbance
Suicidal States, 46, 104, 122, 123, 208
   case studies, 125–126, 126
   with EMDR therapy, 121–126
suicide, 4
sympathetic function, 58–63
Symptom Event Map, 43–44, 97, 102–103, 205–208

TCAs. *See* tricyclics
Teicher, Martin, 9
tolerance, window of, 58–63
touchstone memory, 115
trauma, 9. *See also* attachment trauma
trazodone, 184
TRD. *See* treatment-resistant depression
treatment-resistant depression (TRD), 183–184, 189–190
tricyclics (TCAs), 184
Two Tugs technique, 79

unipolar depression, 4, 100, 172

Validity of Cognition (VOC), 28
verbal abuse, 9
visuo-spatial sketchpad, 29
VOC. *See* Validity of Cognition
vortioxetine, 184

window of tolerance, 58–63
Wolpe, Joseph, 12, 28
working memory hypothesis, 29

yellow light, traffic light, 66, 154

www.ingramcontent.com/pod-product-compliance
Ingram Content Group UK Ltd.
Pitfield, Milton Keynes, MK11 3LW, UK
UKHW021833140426
5217IPUK00021B/1426